Communicating in Hospital Emergency Departments

Diana Slade • Marie Manidis
Jeannette McGregor • Hermine Scheeres
Eloise Chandler • Jane Stein-Parbury
Roger Dunston • Maria Herke
Christian M.I.M. Matthiessen

Communicating in Hospital Emergency Departments

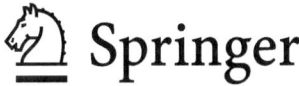

Diana Slade
Marie Manidis
Jeannette McGregor
Hermine Scheeres
Eloise Chandler
Jane Stein-Parbury
Roger Dunston

University of Technology
Sydney
New South Wales
Australia

Maria Herke
Macquarie University
Sydney
New South Wales
Australia

Christian M.I.M. Matthiessen
Hong Kong Polytechnic University
Hong Kong
Hong Kong SAR

ISBN 978-3-662-52457-2   ISBN 978-3-662-46021-4 (eBook)
DOI 10.1007/978-3-662-46021-4

Springer Heidelberg New York Dordrecht London

Printed on acid-free paper

Springer is part of Springer Science+Business Media (www.springer.com)

Preface

This book presents the findings of our research on communication in hospital emergency departments. Our project was conceived in response to the increasing realisation of the central role of communication in effective healthcare delivery, particularly in high stress contexts such as emergency departments (EDs). We present here a detailed picture of the critical importance of communication in the delivery of effective and patient-centred care, and a detailed analysis of the way in which communication occurs and, at times, fails. Failures in communication have consistently been identified as a major cause of critical incidents, that is, adverse events leading to avoidable patient harm. Due to the complex, high stress, unpredictable and dynamic work of EDs, these healthcare environments pose particular challenges for effective communication.

Over a 3-year period, the emergency communication project investigated communication between patients and clinicians[1] (doctors, nurses and allied health professionals) in five representative emergency departments. Combining qualitative ethnographic analysis of the social practices of each ED with discourse analysis of the spoken interactions between clinicians and patients, this project describes the communicative complexity and intensity of work in the ED and, against this backdrop, identifies the features of successful and unsuccessful patient–clinician interactions

In conducting this research, a team of seven researchers with disciplinary backgrounds in applied linguistics and health sciences spent over 1093.5 h inside the

---

[1] Where possible we use the terms 'nurse' or 'doctor' or 'social worker' when it is clear from the context who we are talking about. At other times, this book uses the word 'clinician' to refer inclusively to doctors, nurses, social workers and all the other healthcare professionals/practitioners working in ED. We use the broader term for brevity and simplicity. When referring to a 'junior doctor', we are referring to an intern (JMO, junior medical officer) or resident medical officer (RMO). The term 'registrar' refers to a doctor who is in specialist vocational training. The terms consultant, staff specialist and emergency physician refer to senior medical practitioners with specialist qualifications (e.g. in oncology, neurology, emergency medicine, etc.).

five EDs. Of these hours, 242.75 were spent directly observing ED practices. Eighty-two patient trajectories through the ED were audio recorded and critically analysed, from the patients' first presentations in the ED to the point when a decision was made about their admission, discharge or referral elsewhere. The audio recordings consist of 629,436 words of patient–clinician interactions: affording rich and relevant insights into the links between the overall patient experience and communication practices and breakdowns in the ED. The medical records of each participating patient were also examined and follow-up interviews were conducted with participating patients and staff. In addition, the research team interviewed, and conducted focus groups with, 150 ED staff including administrative staff, nurses and medical practitioners and allied health workers—exploring how these frontline staff perceived the role of, and what they identified as potential barriers to effective, communication within their work. The extensive data collection and the detailed analyses make this one of the most comprehensive studies internationally on clinician–patient communication in hospitals.

The communicative challenges and risks in EDs arise directly from the unique contextual demands of the ED environment. As such, while the focus of this work is on communication, this is integrated with detailed descriptions of the environment, observations, staffing, teamwork and networks of the ED as a means of setting the context for communication encounters.

Communication (whether spoken, gestured, written or electronic) underpins ED practice. From handovers to taking blood, to giving medications, to talking to patients, to listening to colleagues, to reading computer screens, to doing resuscitations—clinicians engage in speaking, listening, reading and writing on a continual basis. The ways the communicative, social and clinical practices work together in the complex context of the ED define the overall quality of the experience for patients and the ultimate work satisfaction of clinicians.

We therefore begin our account of the communication demands by a detailed description of the context of EDs. These contextual factors impact directly on the quality of communication in the ED and pose a series of communicative risks, where information can be lost and patient safety compromised. By presenting a series of vignettes and case studies, we demonstrate the complex communicative networks that exist and illustrate key risk moments within the ED consultation. We then present our analysis of the communication patterns and conventions we observed and recorded: identifying features of effective and ineffective communication.

Our analysis of how clinicians and patients spoke, listened and responded to each other in ED interactions shows that two broad areas of communication have an impact on the quality of the patient journey through the ED:

1. How medical knowledge is communicated.
2. How clinician–patient relationships are established and developed.

We argue that in order to improve the effectiveness of the medical care delivered, clinicians must find more accessible and empathetic ways to communicate medical information and they must establish a more individual, 'human' connection with patients.

In presenting a series of case studies and clear and comparative language examples, we demonstrate how effective patient-centred communication can be achieved within the emergency healthcare context. Drawing on authentic examples of communication patterns within the ED, this book delivers comprehensive communication strategies for the healthcare professional that can be readily imported and integrated into everyday practice.

Diana Slade
Director, Emergency Communication Research
Professor of Applied Linguistics,
Director of the International Research Centre for Communication in Healthcare,
University of Technology Sydney and Hong Kong Polytechnic University
November 2014

Acknowledgements

I would like to thank the cross-disciplinary team of researchers who worked on the project—from the University of Technology Sydney, Marie Manidis, Jeannette McGregor, Hermine Scheeres, Eloise Chandler, Roger Dunston and Nicole Stanton (Faculty of Arts and Social Sciences) and Jane Stein-Parbury (Faculty of Nursing Midwifery and Health); Christian M.I.M. Matthiessen from the Department of English at the Hong Kong Polytechnic University; and Maria Herke from the Linguistics Department, Macquarie University, NSW.

In particular I would like to thank and acknowledge Nicole Staunton who was the project manager for the entire period of the project. Without Nicole this research could not have happened—she was responsible for the administrative organisation of a very complex project. She also undertook many research tasks with great competence.

I would also like to thank Suzanne Eggins and Bernadette Hince from Textwork for their extraordinary editing and layout skills and taking on the job at such short notice.

The team would like to thank all those ED staff and patients who agreed to be interviewed, observed and recorded. At all times staff and patients were remarkably open, prepared to share their experiences, insights and concerns about the work of the ED and, in particular, to discuss the communication that occurs between patients and clinicians. This research study was carried out in collaboration with the staff of the EDs, and in particular with the collaboration of directors of the ED and nursing unit managers. The recommendations were developed in consultation with them.

The rich and authentic recorded data collected as part of the research has enabled us to undertake a unique analysis of the language of ED healthcare. We trust our observations and findings will be useful to ED staff, to hospital management and to patients who attend an emergency department.

We would like to stress that, given the extreme pressures ED staff work under, we were at all times profoundly impressed by their dedication, skill and professionalism—qualities also identified by many patients.

Diana Slade
Director, Emergency Communication Project
Professor of Applied Linguistics, Director of the International Research Centre for
Communication in Healthcare, University of Technology Sydney and Hong Kong
Polytechnic University
November 2014

A Note on Transcription Conventions

We have transcribed clinician–patient interactions using standard English spelling. Nonstandard spellings are occasionally used to capture idiosyncratic or dialectal pronunciations (e.g. *gonna*). Fillers and hesitation markers are transcribed as they are spoken, using the standard English variants, e.g. *Ah, uh huh, hmm, mmm.*

What people say is transcribed without any standardisation or editing. Nonstandard usage is not corrected but transcribed as it was said (e.g. *me feet are frozen*).

Most punctuation marks have the same meaning as in standard written English. Those with special meaning are:

… indicates a trailing off or short hesitation.

==means overlapping or simultaneous talk. For example:

P   Um—oh, just trying to think. Well I suppose you could put my folks down,==yeah.

Z1   == OK, so.

This shows that Z1 started saying *OK, so* when P was saying *yeah.*

— indicates a speaker rephrasing or reworking their contribution, often involving repetition. For example:

P   Ah, no. No, you can take—take him off.

[words in square brackets] are contextual information or information suppressed for privacy reasons. Examples:

[Loud voices in close proximity] contextual information

Z1   And your mobile number I've got [number]. information suppressed

(words in parentheses) were unclear but this is the transcriber's best analysis.

( ) empty parentheses indicate that the transcriber could not hear or guess what was said. For example:

P   Alright then.

Z1   ( ). Transcriber could not hear Z1's comment.

P   OK, thank you very much.

Z1   ( ) *you* ( ). Transcriber could hear only the word *you.*

Contents

List of Figures

List of Tables

Chapter 1
The Role of Communication in Safe and Effective Health Care

1.1 Introduction

Effective communication, both among clinicians and between clinicians and pa-tients, is critical in the provision of safe and quality health care. Over the last two decades, poor communication practices have consistently been identified as a ma-jor cause of critical incidents—adverse events leading to avoidable patient harm—in hospitals around the world (Wilson et al. 1995; Kohn et al. 1999; Hong Kong Hospital Authority 2014; US Joint Commission 2014; NSW Clinical Excellence Commission 2013). The complex, high-stress, unpredictable and dynamic work of emergency departments means that these departments pose particular challenges for effective communication.

In this book, we describe the communicative complexity and intensity of work in emergency departments and, against this backdrop, identify and describe the fea-tures of patient–clinician interactions most likely to lead to patient involvement, patient satisfaction and positive health outcomes. We also detail the communication practices that restrict patient involvement and are susceptible to misunderstandings and breakdowns in communication, which in turn affect patient satisfaction and safety. We then identify ways in which clinicians can enhance their communicative skills to improve the quality and safety of the patient journey through the emergen-cy department. The strategies clinicians use need to simultaneously communicate medical knowledge and build up rapport and empathy with the patient. We argue that to deliver care effectively, clinicians must communicate care effectively.

Conducted in Australia over a 3-year period, our qualitative study investigated communication between patients and clinicians (doctors, nurses and allied health professionals) in five representative emergency departments[1] in New South Wales and the Australian Capital Territory. The study involved 1093 h of observations,

---

[1] Also known throughout the world as Accident & Emergency Departments or Emergency Rooms. Throughout the book we will use the term Emergency Department.

© Springer-Verlag Berlin Heidelberg 2015
D. Slade et al., *Communicating in Hospital Emergency Departments*,
DOI 10.1007/978-3-662-46021-4_1

150 interviews with clinicians and patients, and the audio recording of patient–clinician interactions over the course of 82 patients' emergency department trajectories from triage to disposition. Our research therefore represents one of the most comprehensive studies internationally on patient–clinician communication in hospitals, and specifically within emergency department care. This book documents our research findings, and presents a detailed analysis of the way communication occurs and sometimes fails in the high stress and time-critical context of emergency health care.

Emergency departments are becoming increasingly challenging health care contexts for clinician–patient communication. A defining and universal characteristic of emergency department care is the unpredictability of patient presentations and the lack of familiarity between patients and clinicians. Patients will typically present as strangers to emergency departments, with no readily accessible medical records or established relationships with the clinicians who will be treating them (Hobgood et al. 2002; Chung 2005). As a result, perhaps more than at any other site within the healthcare system, emergency medicine relies heavily on effective spoken communication between patients and clinicians as the former articulate their symptoms and concerns, and the latter draw on this to complement physical examination and diagnosis, and subsequently negotiate treatment (Redfern et al. 2009). Increasing patient demand for emergency department services around the world often results in overcrowding and 'access block' (the inability of a hospital to admit new patients due to a lack of available beds). These pressures have placed severe time constraints on clinician–patient interactions.

It has been recently estimated that the number of presentations to emergency departments increases annually by 3–6 % around the developed world (Lowthian et al. 2012). In England, the National Health Service now estimates that there are over 21 million emergency department attendances each year (National Health Service 2014). The latest statistics published by the US Department of Health and Human Services showed that in 2011, there were more than 131 million presentations to emergency departments in the USA. In Australia, more than 6.7 million emergency department presentations were reported in 2013, representing a 2.5 % increase from the previous year (National Health Performance Authority 2014; Australian Institute of Health and Welfare 2013). This high demand has resulted in emergency departments around the world frequently becoming subject to patient overload, and exceeding staff capacity to provide timely care. This can create serious obstacles to effective clinician–patient communication, obstacles which, if not overcome, can result in serious patient harm.

What is unique about this book is that it studies hospital communications as they unfold. It explains, describes and analyses actual communication between clinicians and patients in real time. The focus is on the patient, and on how the clinician–patient interactions within the emergency department are created, modified and shaped by the complexity of emergency department work. By observing, interviewing and audio recording, we have been able to produce greater insights than would be gained by a single method. Our book is about communication, but we have set the context with descriptions of the environment, observations, staffing, teamwork and networks of the emergency department.

Before we describe the approach we used, we survey significant literature on communication, patient safety and patient-centred care. We also review other research on communication in emergency contexts. A key characteristic of an effective health system is a sensitivity to language and culture in the promotion of health and wellbeing—a patient focused system, delivering patient focused care, communicated in patient sensitive ways (National Public Health Partnership Secretariat 2000). Our motif throughout the book is that communicating care is a core component of delivering care and that due to the unique challenges of the ED context there is a significant gap between patient-centred rhetoric and practice.

1.2   Communication and Patient Safety

Patient safety, defined by the World Health Organization as "freedom … from unnecessary harm or potential harm associated with healthcare" (World Health Organization 2007), is a key and growing concern for health authorities, organisations, clinicians and patients around the world (New South Wales Department of Health 2004; UK Department of Health 2000, 2005; US Institute of Medicine 2001). In 2000, the US Institute of Medicine estimated that between 44,000 and 98,000 patients died in US hospitals annually due to avoidable patient harm. Many of these deaths were attributed to poor communication (Kohn et al. 1999). More recently, in 2013, the number of preventable patient deaths in the USA was revised to be in excess of 400,000 (James 2013). Alongside this, financial costs to governments of avoidable patient harm are also increasing. It has been estimated, for instance, that Australia spends AUD$2 billion a year as a result of avoidable patient harm. One third of this cost is attributed to communication failures (National Health and Hospitals Reform Commission 2008). Poor communication between clinicians and patients has also been repeatedly linked to patients' dissatisfaction with their care, subsequent complaints (Tam and Lau 2000; Lau 2000), and decisions to pursue litigation (Charmel and Frampton 2008; Vincent et al. 1994).

Investigations into patient safety are often approached multidimensionally through studies that gather numerical and statistical data on environmental factors, technical and diagnostic errors, fatigue, pharmacological and surgical mistakes (World Health Organization 2007). Most major health services are thus focused on understanding the most common threats to patient safety from a technical and statistical viewpoint. They investigate the causal nature of clinical incidents (e.g. what failure to carry out a planned action led to patient harm), rather than what happened at a communicative level between clinicians and patients.

Our study arose after a series of government investigations into acute health services in New South Wales. These followed some widely publicised critical incidents in public hospitals (New South Wales Department of Health 2004, 2005). The incidents highlighted the need for systematic, in-depth and *in situ* research into clinician–patient communication practices within public emergency departments. One of the most significant outcomes of the various government investigations was the publication of the findings of the Special Commission of Inquiry into Acute Care Services in NSW Public Hospitals (Garling 2008, Vol. 1).

The Special Commission of Inquiry was launched in the midst of a public outcry following a widely publicised serious incident in a public hospital in NSW. Emergency department clinicians increasingly participated in media interviews in which they described the "chronic" conditions within the emergency department, including extreme understaffing, lack of beds, long shifts, low morale, exhausted staff, lack of supervision of junior doctors and access block (see, e.g. Benson and Smith 2007; Garling 2008, Vol. 1).

The incident that occurred involved, among other factors, communication error and breakdowns, resulting in the death of Vanessa Anderson, a 16 year old schoolgirl. Vanessa had arrived by ambulance at an emergency department, after being struck on the side of the head with a golf ball. She was admitted to hospital, where she died weeks later after suffering a respiratory arrest (Coronial Inquest 2007). In the coronial inquest that followed, Vanessa's death was deemed avoidable—the cumulative result of a series of communication failures between clinicians and between clinicians and Vanessa's family, clinical errors, poorly written records and understaffing. In delivering his findings, the coroner noted that he had never "seen a case such as Vanessa's in which almost every conceivable error or omission was detected and those errors continued to build on top of one another" (Coronial Inquest 2007, p. 14). The coroner called upon the NSW Government to lodge a public inquiry into the delivery of acute health services in NSW. On the day the coroner's findings were delivered, the Premier of NSW announced a Special Commission into Acute Health Services in New South Wales (Garling 2008, Vol. 1).

During submissions to the inquiry, the commission was inundated with patient and carer stories of experiences of unsatisfactory care arising from poor communication between clinicians, patients and their families (Garling 2008, Vol. 2, pp. 551–554). As the commission noted in its final report, failure by clinicians to introduce themselves to patients or their carers and to include patients in discussions of their care were recurrent themes. Indeed, the quality of patient–clinician communication in NSW hospitals based on patient reports was ultimately denounced by the commission as "unacceptable in a civilised society let alone a system of patient centred health care" (Garling 2008, Vol. 2, p. 552). Noting that "healthcare is ultimately about the patient" and that "patients (and their carers) play a key role in ensuring that the healthcare they receive is safe and effective", the commission recommended that greater emphasis be placed on improving clinician–patient communication within all acute health services (Garling 2008, Vol. 2, p. 554). The commission further recommended that far greater efforts be made to provide patients with explanations of emergency department processes, particularly the triage system, and to communicate with patients over the course of their care (Garling 2008, Vol. 2).

1.2.1 Patient-Centred Care

Governments, healthcare organisations, researchers and educators have come to recognise the key role that communication plays in patient safety and the provision of quality health care. This realisation has come with increasing international adoption of a particular model of patient care and communication, known variously as patient-centred care, person-centred care, consumer-centred care, relationship-centred care and client-centred care (McBrien 2009; McCarthy et al. 2013a; McMillan et al. 2013).

Whatever names we give the policy, the main ideas are that patients should be engaged and respected as active and informed participants in their own health care, and that clinicians and healthcare organisations should elicit individual patient preferences, needs and beliefs, and be receptive to these (McBrien 2009; McCarthy et al. 2013a; McMillan et al. 2013; O'Gara and Fairhurst 2004; Pham et al. 2011). Development of effective clinician–patient relationships that balance the clinical focus of healthcare interactions with the development of empathy and rapport between clinicians and patients is essential for patient-centred care (Eggins and Slade 2012; Slade et al. 2008, 2011; Rider et al. 2014; O'Gara and Fairhurst 2004; Hobgood et al. 2002). Improving clinician–patient communication is fundamental— translating medical or clinical discourse and procedures into language that patients can understand, and adopting communication strategies that empower and encourage patients to engage in consultations and make informed decisions about their own health care (Cohen et al. 2013; O'Gara and Fairhurst 2004).

Patient-centred care, and through it patient-centred communication, is increasingly being linked to both patient satisfaction and patient safety. In particular, research has demonstrated the link between patient-centred communication and

- greater levels of patient satisfaction (Ekwall 2013; McMillan et al. 2013; Perez-Carceles et al. 2010),
- engagement in healthcare consultations (McMillan et al. 2013),
- comprehension and understanding of treatment procedures and diagnosis and
- subsequent agreement with clinicians' recommended treatment regimens, and adherence to them (McMillan et al. 2013; Nitzan et al. 2012).

As a result, governments, hospitals and medical and nursing tertiary institutions across the world have now incorporated the language of patient-centred care into their service charters and policies. Patient-centred care is now being posited as the most effective and safe model of healthcare delivery. In Hong Kong, for example, patient-centred care and communication is a goal of the Hong Kong Hospital Authority, the body responsible for the administration and management of public hospitals. In the UK, patient-centred care guides the services of the National Health Service. In Australia, the principles of patient-centred care are in national healthcare strategies and public policy documents, including the Australian Charter of Healthcare Rights and the Australian Safety and Quality Framework for Health Care, and the National Safety and Quality Health Service Standards. All of these emphasise the importance of engaging and respecting patients as informed participants in their health care (Australian Commission on Safety and Quality in Health Care 2011).

The International Research Centre for Communication in Healthcare has developed an International Charter for Human Values in Healthcare (Rider et al. 2014) which details the core values that underpin ethical and safe relationship-centred care. Across the board, patient-centred care is being placed as a benchmark for quality care within all health care contexts.

Despite this widespread policy embrace, to date there has been little research exploring how patient-centred care is being incorporated within the high-stress and time pressured context of emergency departments (McCarthy et al. 2013a). Studies have solicited patient feedback on patient-centred communication styles and information needs (see, for example, Andersson et al. 2014; Buckley et al. 2013; Kington and Short 2010; McCarthy et al. 2013a) and explored emergency department clinician's awareness of the importance and benefits of patient-centred care (Cameron et al. 2010; Cohen et al. 2013; Muntlin et al. 2013). However, very few studies have examined how patient-centred care is enacted in practice (Dale et al. 2008; Dean and Oetzel 2014; Vashi and Rhodes 2011). As McCarthy et al. point out, "patient-centered care remains largely a topic of academic discussion, rather than an integrated part of clinical practice or research in emergency medicine" (McCarthy et al. 2013a, p. 442).

1.3   Communication in Emergency Departments

1.3.1   Research on Patient Experience and Satisfaction

Research on communication in emergency departments has predominantly focused on patient experience surveys or interviews, with very little research describing what actually occurs in spoken interactions between clinicians and patients or in interactions between clinicians about patient care.

Studies of patient experiences in emergency departments have tended to highlight the emotional impact on patients of seeking emergency department care (Gordon et al. 2010). As discussed above, for most patients the emergency department will be unfamiliar territory, not only because of the number of unknown clinicians patients will interact with, but also because of the almost unique organisational procedures and policies they will confront. Over the course of their care, patients will be physically moved throughout the emergency department from the waiting room to a consultation bed, to a prescribed treatment or testing area, and possibly to another hospital ward (Redfern et al. 2009, p. 656). Along the way, they will be asked to share intimate and personal information with a series of medical, nursing and administrative personnel they have never met (O'Gara and Fairhurst 2004, p. 204). As Olthuis and colleagues write:

> For most patients, an emergency department visit means immersion in a culture that is not self evident. The modes of working, the multitude of emergency department staff and their

mutual relations, and the uncommon questions and environments may easily lead to patient concerns. (Olthuis et al. 2014, p. 316)

Common themes that have emerged in research exploring patient experiences of emergency department care include feelings of bewilderment, loss of control, anxiety, frustration and prolonged and unexplained waiting times (Olthuis et al. 2014, p. 316; O'Gara and Fairhurst 2004, p. 204).

Other studies of patient experiences and preferences have reinforced the link between the incorporation of patient-centred communication styles and patient satisfaction in the emergency department context. They have particularly highlighted the importance of clinicians providing ongoing information to patients about all aspects of their emergency department care, to help alleviate patient anxiety, allow for greater comprehension of the emergency department processes and patients' illness and equip patients with a sense of control over their health care (see Frank et al. 2009; Elmqvist et al. 2011; Kington and Short 2010, p. 408). In turn, research focusing on clinician perspectives has shown an increased awareness of the benefits of incorporating patient-centred strategies in securing better patient outcomes.

However, these studies have also emphasised that for many emergency department clinicians, providing patient-centred care is often seen to be in conflict with the time-pressured environment. While clinicians may be aware of its benefits, the literature suggests that patient-centred care continues to be regarded as a desirable add-on, rather than a core component of emergency department practice. Indeed, although small in number, studies that have examined clinician–patient interactions in the emergency department have shown a tendency among emergency department clinicians to maintain tight control over their conversations with patients, often at the expense of developing rapport, ensuring patient comprehension of explanations and enabling patient participation (Slade et al. 2008). Notably, however, when patient-centred communication styles were implemented by emergency department clinicians, they were not found to lengthen patient-clinician consultations (McMillan et al. 2013, p. 592; Rhodes et al 2004).

In the most recently published patient satisfaction survey conducted by NSW Health, non-admitted emergency patients "were the least likely to report that their care had been well explained" to them (NSW Health 2012, p. 23). Fifty eight per cent of the respondents assessed the explanations clinicians had given them positively, 25 % were neutral and 17 % were negative (NSW Health 2012, p. 23). Patient satisfaction surveys, while important, do not provide adequate measures of patient comprehension of diagnosis or treatment plans—key elements in patient health outcomes once they leave emergency departments.

Follow-up studies carried out internationally have shown that even positive assessments of a clinician's information-giving practices by patients do not correlate with patients' comprehension levels and subsequent abilities to adhere appropriately to recommended treatment regimens following their discharge (Crane 1997; Engel et al. 2009; Gignon et al. 2013). Patient comprehension of a diagnosis and of how to treat their condition is essential for effective health outcomes, including patient satisfaction and treatment adherence (Clancy 2009) and ability to seek and access follow-up care (Alberti and Nannini 2013). It also serves "as a meaningful measure of what patient takes away from their visit and thereby provides a valuable tool for communication research" (Engel et al. 2009, p. 459).

Other research in emergency departments has shown correlations between effective clinician–patient communication and positive patient outcomes. Benefits include greater rates of patient satisfaction (see, e.g. Ekwall 2013; McMillan et al. 2013, p. 586; Perez-Carceles et al. 2010, p. 459); parallel decreases in patient complaints and litigation (see, e.g. Charmel and Frampton 2008; Lau 2000); higher levels of patient comprehension of diagnosis and treatment and subsequent adherence to hospital discharge or treatment instructions (see, e.g. McMillan et al. 2013; Nitzan et al. 2012); and declines in rates of rehospitalisation (Clancy 2009; Jack et al. 2009).

In interviews and surveys many emergency department clinicians have reported that there is not sufficient time to develop rapport and empathy with a patient (see Chandler et al., in preparation). However, our research and other studies have shown that, when patient-centred communication styles were implemented by emergency department clinicians, they were not found to lengthen patient–clinician consultations (McMillan et al. 2013, p. 592; Rhodes et al. 2004).

A large proportion of patient-centred care research in emergency departments has been in the form of patient experience surveys. These are *quantitatively* driven, angled at delivering statistical overviews of patient and clinician experiences, preferences and levels of awareness of the benefits of adopting patient-centred communication styles. Patient satisfaction surveys have been a particularly prominent tool for assessing patient experiences of emergency care, and their preferences and needs (Nairn et al. 2004, p. 161). These have provided large-scale overviews of what patients value in their interactions with emergency department clinicians, as well as suggesting shortcomings in clinician information-giving and interpersonal communication practices.

More recently, there has been a move to assess the *quality* and presence of patient-centred care in emergency departments by testing levels of patient satisfaction with specific tenets of patient-centred care. For example, a recent study by McCarthy and colleagues (McCarthy et al. 2013b) asked patients to rate their experiences of clinician communication styles immediately following their discharge from the emergency department. Items that were included related to patient-centred communication styles including the extent to which patients felt they were given the time to describe what concerned them, the quality of a clinician's explanations, displays of empathy by clinicians, and whether patients were encouraged to ask questions and participate in decision-making. Nearly three quarters of the patient respondents rated the following items as excellent:

- Letting the patient talk without interruptions
- Talking in terms that patients could understand
- Treating the patient with respect and showing care and concern

The lowest ratings were given to these factors which are equally fundamental to patient-centred care:

- Clinicians encouraging patients to ask questions
- Greeting patients in a way that made them feel comfortable
- Involving patients in decision-making
- Showing interest in patients' ideas about their own health (McCarthy et al. 2013a, p. 265)

Although such studies provide large-scale overviews of what patients value and experience in interactions with emergency department clinicians, it can be argued that their predominantly quantitative approach, angled at producing statistical data, does not allow for an in-depth or nuanced exploration of respondent experiences. Rather, their typical closed question and tick-the-box answer form reduces patient responses to a series of predetermined statements, rather than as Nairn et al. point out "elicit[ing] [the] inherent complexity" of the patient experience" (Nairn et al. 2004, p. 163).

1.3.2 Research into Communication Practices in Emergency Departments

Researchers have only recently begun to examine actual communication practices that occur within emergency departments. Early social science approaches to clinical communication focused mainly on general practice, foregrounding medical communication in primary care settings, and neglecting the dynamic features of communication within the more multidisciplinary and time-pressured acute care settings.

Over the last three years, there has been a move by researchers to examine emergency department patient–clinician communication through observations or recorded segments of consultations rather than just through surveys and interviews. Although studies are small in number, they have been predominantly quantitatively driven and geared towards exploring correlations between the informational content of emergency department discharge conversations and patient comprehension and adherence once they leave (see, e.g. Coleman et al. 2013; Nitzan et al. 2012; Gignon et al. 2013).

The discharge conversation, when it occurs, represents the final opportunity in the acute patient's journey to discuss their diagnosis, test results and planned follow-up care (including medication prescriptions and dosages) (Vashi and Rhodes 2011, p. 316). Research to date has linked communication failures at this point (commonly defined within the literature as inadequate information-giving on the clinician's behalf and subsequent lack of patient comprehension of discharge instructions) to non-adherence with treatment plans and subsequent adverse events, leading to rehospitalisation (Buckley et al. 2013, p. 1–2). As Clancy writes, without effective clinician–patient communication before a patient's departure from hospital, patients run the risk of being "unprepared to care for themselves or to know how or when to seek follow-up care" (Clancy 2009, p. 344). When patients understand their diagnosis and how to monitor and treat themselves (including comprehending the reasons for recommended treatment plans), they are more likely to adhere to the recommended treatment regimen and have better perceptions of the quality of care received (see, e.g. Crane 1997, p. 4; Coleman et al. 2013).

In fact, recent studies indicate that a patient's understanding of these is far more likely to predict adherence and patient safety following discharge than other factors such as their age, education level and even diagnosis (see, e.g. Nitzan et al. 2012). Such findings have led some to argue that securing patient's understanding of their condition and treatment before their discharge "is not only important from the perspective of patients' rights but is valuable clinically" (Nitzan et al. 2012, p. 115). There is now growing evidence that even when the clinician responsible for discharge has provided information to the patient summarising the diagnosis, exams already performed, treatment follow-up plans and prescribed medication, this will not necessarily translate to adequate levels of patient understanding and subsequent ability to comply with the follow-up instructions after their departure from the clinician's care (see Samuels-Kalow et al. 2011, p. 153). As Marty et al. argue, "it is not the information communicated but the information understood that is the decisive factor for patient compliance" (Marty et al. 2013, p. 53).

Current research on emergency department discharge processes suggests that discharge conversations tend to be fragmented, variable and incomplete (Marty et al. 2013, p. 53) or as Samuels-Kalow et al. (2011, p. 152) put it, an "afterthought". While the discharge conversation provides a final opportunity for patient education, it is only one part of the ongoing patient–clinician dialogue throughout the emergency department patient's journey. Vashi and Rhodes argue that research that does not examine the patient throughout the entire emergency department visit may miss integral points of clinician–patient information exchange, and important discourse features which may be crucial to patient comprehension, compliance and safety behaviour post emergency department discharge (Vashi and Rhodes 2011, p. 315).

In the present research, we have observed and recorded the entire patient journey through the hospital from triage to disposition. It was beyond the scope of this research to follow the patient after discharge but we argue in the final chapter that researching the patient's continuity of care from discharge to the community is an important complement to this research. A team led by Phillip Della and involving among others Diana Slade and Roger Dunstan has just started an extensive project in Australia, following three vulnerable groups of patients—the elderly, mental health and paediatric—from the point of discharge to the community. The aim of this project is to improve patient safety outcomes by analysing and then enhancing communication practices during transition of care at discharge for high risk clinical populations.

1.4 Our Qualitative Approach

Understanding the context of emergency departments is an essential prerequisite for understanding and describing the communication in that context. Our research combined two complementary modes of qualitative analysis: discourse[2] analysis of authentic interactions between clinicians (nurses, doctors and allied health workers) and patients; and qualitative ethnographic analysis of the social, organisational, and interdisciplinary clinician practices of each emergency department. The combination of these two approaches allowed us to comprehensively describe and analyse the dynamics of patient–clinician communication in emergency departments. It provided insights into how the emergency department context affects clinician communication practices, and how these practices shape patient and clinician experiences and perspectives of emergency care. Our approach was enhanced and enriched by the fact that the research team consisted of professionals with expertise in linguistics, medicine, nursing, allied health, health policy and communication studies, applying both insider and outsider perspectives to how institutional practices and relationships are enacted and realised in particular communication patterns.

1.4.1 Data Collection

The data were collected in the following ways:

- In all, 1095 hrs of non-participant observations were conducted across the five emergency departments, with more than 240 hrs of direct observations.
- Interviews were conducted with 150 emergency department staff (administrative personnel, nurses, doctors, allied health workers).
- Audio recordings were made of 82 patient journeys through the emergency department, capturing all interactions that occurred between the patient and their attending clinicians, or other emergency department or hospital staff, from triage (assessed and categorised for emergency care) to the time of their disposition (when a decision was made either to admit them or send them home). The 82 patient journey recordings totalled 1,411,238 transcribed words. This represents

---

[2] At its simplest level, "discourse" is any meaningful stretch of language. It can be as brief as "Look out" (which means something particular if one is in immediate danger) or an extended stretch of talk, such as one full consultation that we have recorded. "Discourse analysis" focuses on describing the structure and function of naturally occurring spoken language (see Eggins and Slade 1997). In this book we examine, for example, how clinicians use language: what terms they use; what positions or stances they adopt through their language and how these position patients/others. In an institutional context, 'discourses differ with the kinds of institutions and social practices in which they take shape and with the positions of those who speak and those whom they address' (ibid.). Thus, a discourse is not a disembodied collection of statements, but groupings of utterances or sentences, statements which are enacted within a social context, which are determined by that social context and which contribute to the way that social context continues its existence" (Macdonnell, 1986, cited in Mills, 1997/2001: p10–11).

one of the largest corpora internationally of actual patient–clinician communication in hospital contexts.

Participant consent was obtained first verbally and then in writing. Only patients in triage categories 3, 4 and 5 were approached. Patients with immediate or imminent life-threatening conditions (triage categories 1 and 2) were not approached. Participant confidentiality was an important feature at all stages of data collection and analysis. Patient and clinician identities have been strictly protected. Strict ethical guidelines have been adhered to in the collection, storage, analysis and discussion of data throughout the research. The record of the interactions as they actually occurred *in situ* provides a unique resource that enables rich and relevant insights into the links between the overall patient experience and communication practices and breakdowns in the emergency department. Our ethnographic approach involved situating the patient experiences and communication exchanges within the professional and institutional practices of each emergency department. The researchers immersed themselves in the context of each emergency department by observing and interviewing key staff and patients. This approach provided a backdrop for understanding the subsequent recorded interactions between clinicians and patients. The recorded patient–clinician interactions were transcribed and analysed in detail (see "A note on transcription conventions" at the beginning of the book).

A distinctive feature of our qualitative methodology is that it uses theoretically consistent, complementary methods to provide a multifaceted and detailed analysis of emergency department communicative practice. Data from each of the phases—the observational data, the interviews and the audio-recordings—were triangulated in the analysis in order to produce greater insight than would be gained by a single method. The value of using qualitative approaches in health communication research has been widely discussed in the literature. As Kuper et al. (2008, p. 406) note, "Qualitative methods are…increasingly prevalent in medical and related research. They provide additional ways for health researchers to explore and explain the contexts in which they and their patients function, enabling a more comprehensive understanding of many aspects of the healthcare system".

For a detailed account of communication practices in emergency departments, and the relationship between these and the quality and safety of the patient experience, a qualitative approach yields much richer data than a purely quantitative approach. Qualitative studies allow you to explore why and how. As Sullivan et al. (2011, p. 449) say,

> Qualitative approaches are used when the potential answer to a question requires an explanation, not a straightforward yes/no. Generally, qualitative research is concerned with cases rather than variables, and understanding differences rather than calculating the mean of responses … A qualitative study is concerned with the point of view of the individual under study.

Below we describe our ethnographic approach, before outlining how we analyse the spoken interactions.

1.4.2 Methods

1.4.2.1 Ethnographic Analysis

Our ethnographic approach involved situating patient experiences and communication exchanges within the professional and institutional practices of each emergency department. It involved extensive non-participant observations across the various sites within each emergency department (the waiting room, consultations rooms, treatment areas), participant observations through shadowing of clinicians (managerial, medical and nursing), semi-structured interviews with emergency department management, senior and junior medical and nursing staff, and patients; and photographs of signage, written notices and informal notes observed in each emergency department. These ethnographic methods provided a backdrop for understanding the recorded interactions between patients and clinicians.

Non-participant Observation of the Emergency Departments

We recorded what we observed in the emergency departments using observation sheets that could document both structured observational information and general commentary and description—what happened to patients, bedside practices, the work of clinicians (their interactions with each other and with patients), particular events and the layout of the spaces. We observed and noted what clinicians, patients, organisational staff and carers were doing and saying during the time of care, where they were located and who they spoke to. Our observation notes included how the clinician and patient interactions in the emergency department context were created and modified. We observed and noted differences in the ways the nurses and doctors communicated with the patients, differences in communicative style between the senior and junior doctors and between junior and senior nurses, and the way that the patient was positioned in the interactions. We analysed this data inductively with field notes and combined it with the analysis of the interview data. We identified and explored the different factors that affected the patient experience and health outcomes.

Participant Observation Through Clinician Shadowing

We followed a number of clinicians throughout their shifts, audio recording their interactions with patients, other clinicians and management. During this process, we conducted impromptu field interviews with participating clinicians to seek clarification and explanation of observed interactions and activities (Nugus and Braithwaite 2010, p. 513). The audio recordings of clinician shadowing were transcribed in full.

Semi-structured Interviews and Focus Groups with Key Clinical Staff

We conducted semi-structured interviews with key informants (clinicians, hospital and emergency department managers and relevant administrative staff) to get an overall picture of the numbers and types of interactions, problems and issues related to communication, and the clinical and communicative 'traffic' of the emergency department. We also focused on themes and issues in relation to communication; how work and care were organised; how clinicians saw their professional roles and how they spoke about their practices. All interviews were recorded and transcribed verbatim.

Semi-structured Interviews with Patients

We conducted semi-structured interviews with the patients whose emergency department journeys were recorded. These interviews took place following their discharge from the emergency department and were recorded with the patient's consent. We explored a loose set of questions but allowed the interviewers to reorient the interview to follow up on interviewees' responses.

1.4.2.2   Discourse Analysis of the Patient's Journey Through the Emergency Department

As emergency medicine is dominated by spoken language, our focus was on the analysis and description of the spoken interactions with and around the patient. The spoken language was analysed for discourse and grammatical features. By "discourse", we mean any stretch of spoken or written language that is meaningful within its context of use. Discourse features include how explanations and instructions are given and how they are received and acknowledged; how information is sought and clarified; how disputes and differences are negotiated; how breakdowns are repaired; and how empathy and rapport are displayed. From this analysis we were able to develop explanations for the forms of talk used by participants in the context of the emergency department.

We drew on functional approaches to discourse analysis and language description. The overall frameworks for analysis were the theoretical perspectives of sociolinguistics (Gumperz 1982) and systemic functional linguistics (Halliday and Matthiessen 2004; Eggins and Slade 2006). Once patients had consented, all their interactions with clinicians were audio recorded. We transcribed these clinician–patient interactions in detail, checked them for accuracy, and then analysed them linguistically to determine, among other features:

- The functions and language patterns of different stages of the patient journeys through the emergency department, what we refer to in Chap. 3 as the "activity stages"
- The functions and language patterns of the different stages of the actual doctor–patient consultations, what we refer to as the generic stages

- How patients and clinicians exchanged information, including how clinicians communicated medical information (Chap. 5) while building an interpersonal relationship with the patient (Chap. 6)
- How diagnoses were delivered and treatment plans explained and comprehended
- Characteristic features of different disciplinary discourses, for example, the different interactive styles of talk for nurses and doctors
- Differences in styles of clinician communication with patients according to level of seniority, for example, ways junior doctors elicit relevant medical information from patients compared to how senior, more experienced doctors do, and to what extent, if any, this affects the patient experience
- How (or whether) patients understood what was happening to them during their stay in the emergency department

1.4.3   Research Sites

The research was conducted in five public hospital emergency departments, four in New South Wales and one in the Australian Capital Territory. All research sites were teaching hospitals affiliated with university medical schools. In each, the patient demography varied, with presentations by patients from different socioeconomic, cultural and linguistic backgrounds, reflective of multicultural Australia. We will now briefly describe each research site. Table 1.1 summarises the key comparative information about each site.

1.4.3.1   Hospital A

Located in urban Sydney, at the time of research Hospital A provided a number of differentiated emergency care services including an acute, subacute and emergency medicine unit (EMU) facility; a psychiatric emergency care centre; and three resuscitation beds.

During our data collection period (spanning 4 months), the emergency department was providing treatment to approximately 130 patients a day. We audio recorded and observed 19 patients' journeys, conducted semi-structured interviews with 30 clinicians and carried out an additional 65 hrs of observations here. Of the patients we audio recorded, three were over 80 years of age, one was over 70, three were in their 60s, two in their 50s, four were over 40, three over 30 and three were in their 20s. All were English speakers. Several had immigrated to Australia from countries including Sri Lanka, Croatia, Spain, the UK, Lebanon and Iran.

Table 1.1 Comparative data for the five emergency departments studied

	Hospital A	Hospital B	Hospital C	Hospital D	Hospital E
Number of presentations annually (figures provided by each hospital)	44,791	29,908	49,916	56,198	59,017
Average number of patients seen per day in time we were at the hospital	120	81	137.6	151	134 a day on average in 2006 160 a day on average in 2009 (19% increase)
Triage category as % of presentations (in 2008–09)	cat 1 1.2% cat 2 6.9% cat 3 40.2% cat 4 42.0% cat 5 9.6%	cat 1 0.3% cat 2 7.7% cat 3 23.1% cat 4 47.9% cat 5 20.9%	cat 1 0.4% cat 2 8.9% cat 3 30.6% cat 4 50.3% cat 5 9.8%	cat 1 0.6% cat 2 13.4% cat 3 34.8% cat 4 42.4% cat 5 8.8%	cat 1 1.5% cat 2 11.8% cat 3 37.9% cat 4 43.8% cat 5 5.0%
Patient demographic	Mixed ethnicity; high drug and alcohol presentations; inner city; no trauma	Mixed ethnicity; suburban; English speaking background and elderly	Elderly; English speaking background, trauma; suburban	Mixed demographic; younger population than other emergency departments	Culturally diverse family population plus elderly English speaking background patients

1.4.3.2   Hospital B

Hospital B, located in a suburban area in northern Sydney, was not a major trauma emergency department, so patients with very serious injuries are frequently diverted to another emergency department within the broader geographic area. It does, however, provide wide ranging services to its community including a "fast track" option for more straightforward patient presentations where no treatment is required (e.g. a change of bandages); a trainee nurse practitioner service; and an acute and subacute facility. It has two resuscitation beds. There is a psychiatric emergency care centre very close by.

During our data collection period, the emergency department treated 61–100 patients a day. While the patient demography varied in terms of linguistic backgrounds and age, a proportionately large number of elderly patients with multiple co-morbidities presented to this emergency department, many of whom were of an English-speaking background. Our data collection reflects this elderly demographic: of the 17 patient journeys we audio recorded there, four patients were over 80 years old and seven over 60. Ten were female and seven male. We interviewed 20 clinicians, and spent just over 20 hrs carrying out observations.

1.4.3.3   Hospital C

Located in a major regional hub in New South Wales, at the time of research Hospital C provided the full range of emergency department services, including a fast track option, an acute and subacute facility, and three resuscitation beds. A mental health team is also based within the department.

During the time of our data collection, it was estimated that 120–137 patients presented to this emergency department each day, with 12,666 presentations in the 3 months when we conducted our data collection. Like Hospital B, a large proportion of this emergency department's patients were over 65 years of age. At the time of research, 67 % of patients were above 60 years, 31 % were in their 60s, 23 % in their 70s and 13 % over 80. Almost all were born in Australia and were of an English-speaking background. At Hospital C, we audio recorded 15 patients' journeys, interviewed 37 clinicians and spent just over 42 hrs carrying out observations. Of the patients we followed, three were over 80 years in age, eight were over 60, two were over 50 and three were under 50. All were native English speakers.

1.4.3.4   Hospital D

At the time of research, Hospital D, the major public hospital in the Australian Capital Territory, was a teaching hospital for one of the major medical schools in the region. The emergency department provided a fast track option; a nurse practitioner service; an acute, subacute and EMU facility; provision for mental health patients; and three resuscitation beds. During our data collection period, the emergency department received an average of 151 patient presentations each day. The patient de-

Table 1.2 Summary of data collected at the five research sites

Hospital	A	B	C	D	E	Total
Patients per day	130	61–100	120–137	151	134–162	n/a
Patient journeys recorded	19	17	15	19	12	82
Total word count	387,256 words	318,436 words	182,522 words	135,768 words	387,256 words	1,411,238 words
Staff interviews	30	20	37	34	29	150
Direct observations	65 hrs	20 hrs	42 hrs	47 hrs	67 hrs	241 hrs
Total time in emergency department	294 hrs	196 hrs	215 hrs	237½ hrs	151 hrs	1093½ hrs

mography varied, although once more most were born in Australia and were native English speakers. We recorded 19 patient journeys in this emergency department, and interviewed 34 clinicians. We also conducted 47 hrs of observations. Of the patients we followed, one was over 85, two were over 70, two were over 60, three were over 50, four were over 40, three were over 30 and four were in their 20s. All but three were native English-speakers.

1.4.3.5   Hospital E

This emergency department was one of the busiest emergency departments in New South Wales and the major trauma centre for southern Sydney at the time of research. It provided a number of differentiated emergency care services including a fast track option; an acute, subacute and EMU facility; a nurse practitioner; a psychiatric emergency care centre; and three resuscitation beds. During the period we conducted our research here, the hospital received 59,017 trauma presentations. Twenty per cent of these trauma patients were less than 16 years of age. We conducted two rounds of data collection here, over a period of 3 years. During that time, the number of emergency department presentations increased by 19%. Of the patients we audio recorded, one patient was in their 20s, four were in their 30s, three were over 40 and five were over 80. All were English speakers. In addition, 29 clinicians were interviewed and over 67 hrs of observations were conducted.

Table 1.2 summarises the data collected from each of five hospitals.

1.5   Conclusion

Communication (whether spoken, gestured, written or electronic) underpins emergency department practice. From handovers to taking blood, giving medications, talking to patients, listening to colleagues, reading computer screens, and doing resuscitations, clinicians engage in speaking, listening, reading and writing on a continual basis. The ways the communicative, social and clinical practices work together in the complex context of the emergency department define the overall quality of the experience for patients and the ultimate work satisfaction of clinicians. The communicative challenges and risks in emergency departments arise directly from the unique contextual demands of the environment. While the focus of our book is communication, we have integrated this with descriptions of the environment, observations, staffing, teamwork and networks of the emergency department as a means of setting the context for the communicative interactions.

The book therefore offers a systemic and information-rich description and analysis of the complex communication ecology of contemporary emergency departments. The study's uniqueness lies in its approach: patients have been observed and recorded in conversation with healthcare practitioners and administration staff from the moment they enter the emergency department (at "triage") until the moment a decision is made about treatment ("disposition") or release from the emergency department. Our analytic framing has developed an approach to emergency department practice that suggests areas of communicative vulnerability, identifying risk and practices that either increase or diminish risk. Encounters are located within the complex and institutionally governed frameworks of social interactions, relationships and situations specific to the emergency department and the hospital in question.

We consider the 'taken for granted' language and communication networks of clinicians in the emergency department and we examine them closely. That is, by focusing on the authentic language and communication practices used in the consultations, we analyse the following communicative dimensions:

- How misunderstandings arise
- How clinicians question patients
- How medical terminology is used with patients
- How diagnoses are shared with patients
- How clinicians relay important information to the patient
- What novice practitioners and their more senior counterparts say, how they say it, and to whom they say it
- How the language choices and communication network practices of clinicians and patients can potentially risk patient safety and how this potential risk is negotiated or avoided

We begin this book by providing an overview of the emergency department context, exploring the ways in which the emergency department's unique context becomes reflected in particular communication practices between patients and clinicians (Chap. 2).

Drawing on our ethnographic data, we then describe key features of the emergency department patient's journey from triage to admission, outlining how the patient's trajectory becomes organised into four distinct stages: triage, nursing admission, initial medical consultation (initial contact, exploration of condition, history-taking, diagnostic tests and procedures) and the final medical consultation consisting of diagnosis, treatment and disposition (Chap. 3). This fragmentation into stages directly affects the quality of communication in the emergency department and poses a series of moments which act as communicative risks, where information can be lost and patient safety compromised.

By presenting a series of transcripts of actual interactions we illustrate key risk moments within the emergency department consultation that have the potential to affect patient safety. We have coined the term "potential risk points" to describe the moments in the interactions between the clinician and the patient where misalignments or misunderstandings take place—that cumulatively affect the quality of the patient experience and potentially patient safety (Chap. 4).

In Chaps. 5 and 6 we continue our detailed description of the communication, focusing on the clinician–patient consultations by outlining the key communication strategies clinicians can use for effectively communicating medical knowledge and information (Chap. 5) and interpersonal strategies they can use to effectively involve patients in their care (Chap. 6). In Chap. 7, we outline action strategies for improving communication in emergency departments.

References

Alberti, T., & Nannini, A. (2013). Patient comprehension of discharge instructions from the emergency department: A literature review. *Journal of the American Association of Nurse Practitioners, 25*, 186–194.

Andersson, H., Wireklint, B. S., Nilsson, K., & Jakobsson, E. (2014). Management of everyday work in emergency departments—An exploratory study with Swedish managers. *International Emergency Nursing, 22*(4), 190–196.

Australian Commission on Safety and Quality in Health Care (2011). *Patient-centred care: Improving quality and safety through partnerships with patients and consumers*. Sydney: ACSQHC.

Australian Institute of Health and Welfare (2013). *Australian hospital statistics 2012–13: Emergency department care*. Canberra: AIHW.

Benson, K., & Smith, A. (2007, September 27). Birth in toilet in hospital without care. *Sydney Morning Herald*.

Buckley, B., McCarthy, D., Forth, V., Tanabe, P., Schmidt, M., Adams, J., Engel, K. (2013). Patient input into the development and enhancement of emergency department discharge instructions: A focus group study. *Journal of Emergency Nursing, 39*(6), 553–561.

Cameron, K. A., Engel, K. G., McCarthy, D. M., Buckley, B. A., Kollar, L. M. M., Donlan, S. M., Pang, P. S., Makoul, G., Tanabe, P., Gisondi, M. A., & Adams, J. G. (2010). Examining emergency department communication through a staff-based participatory research method: Identifying barriers and solutions to meaningful change. *Annals of Emergency Medicine, 56*(6), 614–622.

Charmel, P., & Frampton, S. (2008). Building the business case for patient-centred care. *Healthcare Financial Management, 62*(3), 80–85.

Chung, C. (2005). Meeting the challenges of rising patient expectations: The 10 "C"s for emergency physicians. *Hong Kong Journal of Emergency Medicine, 12*, 3–5.

Clancy, C. (2009). Reengineering hospital discharge: A protocol to improve patient safety, reduce costs and boost patient satisfaction. *American Journal of Medical Quality, 24*, 344–346.

Cohen, E., Wilken, H., Tannebaum, M., Plew, M., Haley, L. Jr. (2013). When patients are impatient: The communication strategies utilised by emergency department employees to manage patients frustrated by wait times. *Health Communication, 28*(3), 275–285.

Coleman, E., Chugh, A., Williams, M., Grigsby, J., Glasheen, J., McKenzie, M., & Min, S.J. (2013). Understanding and execution of discharge instructions. *American Journal of Medical Quality, 28*(5), 383–391.

Coronial Inquest. (2007). Inquest into the death of Vanessa Anderson by Milovanovich C, Magistrate (NSW Deputy State Coroner). Westmead file. No. 161/2007. Sydney: Westmead Coroner's Court, 24 Jan 2008.

Crane, J. (1997). Patient comprehension of doctor-patient communication of discharge from the emergency department. *Journal of Emergency Medicine, 15*(1), 1–7.

Dale, J., Sandhu, H., Lall, R., & Glucksman, E. (2008). The patient, the doctor and the emergency department: A cross-sectional study of patient-centredness in 1990 and 2005. *Patient Education and Counseling, 72*, 320–329.

Dean, M., & Oetzel, J. G. (2014). Physicians' perspectives of managing tensions around dimensions of effective communication in the emergency department. *Health Communication, 29*(3), 257–266.

Eggins, S., & Slade, D. (2006, first published 1997). *Analysing casual conversation.* London: Equinox.

Eggins, S., & Slade, D. (2012). Clinical handover as an interactive event: Informational and interactional communication strategies in effective shift-change handovers. *Communication & Medicine, 9*(3), 215–227.

Ekwall, A. (2013). Acuity and anxiety from the patient's perspective in the emergency department. *Journal of Emergency Nursing, 39*, 534–548. doi:10.1016/j.jen.2010.10.003.

Elmqvist C., Fridlund, B., Ekebergh, M. (2011). On a hidden game board: The patient's first encounter with emergency care at the emergency department. *Journal of Clinical Nursing, 21*, 17–18.

Engel K. G., Heisler, M., Smith, D. M., Robinson, C. H., Forman, J. H., & Ubel, P. A. (2009). Patient comprehension of emergency department care and instructions: Are patients aware of when they do not understand? *Annals of Emergency Medicine, 53*(4), 454–461.

Frank, C., Asp, M., & Dahlberg, K. (2009). Patient participation in emergency care—A phenomenographic analysis of caregivers' conceptions. *Journal of Clinical Medicine, 18*(18), 2555–2562.

Garling, P. (2008). *Final report of the Special commission of inquiry: Acute care services in NSW public hospitals* (Vol. 1–2). Sydney: Special Commission of Inquiry.

Gignon, M., Ammirati, C., Mercier, R., & Detave, M. (2013). Compliance with emergency department discharge instructions. *Journal of Emergency Nursing, 40*(1), 51–55.

Gordon, J., Shepherd, L. A., & Anaf, S. (2010). The patient experience in the emergency department: A systematic synthesis of qualitative research. *International Emergency Nursing, 18*, 80–88.

Gumperz, J.J. (1982). *Discourse strategies.* London: Cambridge University Press.

Halliday, M. A. K., & Matthiessen, C. M. I. M. (2004). *An introduction to functional grammar* (3rd ed.). London: Edward Arnold.

Hobgood, C., Riviello, R., Jourilles, N., & Hamilton, G. (2002). Assessment of communication and interpersonal skills competencies. *Academic Emergency Medicine, 9*(11), 1257–1268.

Hong Kong Hospital Authority (2014). Annual report on sentinel and serious untoward events: 1 October 2012–30 September 2013. http://www.ha.org.hk/haho/ho/psrm/ECOPYSEREPORT2014.PDF. Accessed 29 March 2014.

Jack, B., Chetty, V., Anthony, D., Greenwald, J., Sanchez, G., Johnson, A., Forsythe, S., O'Donnell, J., Passche-Orlow, M., Manasseh, C., Martin, S., & Culpepper, L. (2009). A re-engineered hospital discharge program to decrease re-hospitalisation. *Annals of Internal Medicine, 150*, 178–187.

James, J. (2013). A new, evidence-based estimate of patient harms associated with hospital care. *Journal of Patient Safety, 9*(3), 122–128.

Kington, M., & Short, A. (2010). What do consumers want to know in the emergency department? *International Journal of Nursing Practice, 16*, 406–411.

Kohn, L. T., Corrigan, J. M., & Donaldson, M. S. (1999). *To err is human: Building a safer health system*. Washington DC: National Academy Press.

Kuper, A., Reeves, S., & Levinson, W. (2008). An introduction to reading and appraising qualitative research. *BMJ, 337*, 404–407.

Lau, F. L. (2000). Can communication skills workshops for emergency department doctors improve patient satisfaction? *Emergency Medicine Journal, 17*, 251–253.

Lowthian, J., Curtis, A., Jolley, D., Stoelwinder, J., McNeil, J., & Cameron, P. (2012). Demand at the emergency department front door: 10-year trends in presentations. *Medical Journal of Australia, 196*(2), 128–132.

Marty, H., Bogenstatter, Y., Franc, G., Tschan, F., & Simmerman, H. (2013). How well informed are patients when leaving the emergency department? Comparing information provided and information retained. *Emergency Medicine Journal, 30*, 53–57.

McBrien, B. (2009). Translating change: The development of a person-centred triage training programme for emergency nurses'. *International Emergency Nursing, 17*, 31–37.

McCarthy, D., Buckley, B., Engel, K., Foth, V., Adams, J., & Cameron, K. (2013a). Understanding patient-provider conversation: What are we talking about? *Academic Emergency Medicine, 20*(5), 441–448.

McCarthy, D., Ellison, E. P., Venkatesh, A. K., Engle, K. G., Camoron, K. A., Makoul, G., & Adams, J. (2013b). Emergency department team communication with the patient: The patient's perspective. *Journal of Medicine, 45*(2), 262–270.

McMillan, S., Kendall, E., Sav, A., King, M., Whitty, J., Kelly, F., & Wheeler, A. (2013). Patient-centred approaches to healthcare: A systematic review of randomised controlled trials. *Medical Care Research and Review, 70*, 567–596.

Muntlin, A., Carlsson, M., & Gunningberg, L. (2013). Barriers to change hindering quality improvement: The reality of emergency care. Journal of Emergency Nursing, *36*(4), 317–323.

Nairn, S., Whotton, E., Marsal, C., Roberts, M., & Swann, G. (2004). The patient experience in emergency departments: A review of the literature. *Accident & Emergency Nursing, 12*, 159–165.

National Health and Hospitals Reform Commission. (2008). *Beyond the blame game: Accountability and performance benchmarks for the next Australian health care agreements*. Canberra: National Health & Hospitals Reform Commissions. http://www.health.gov.au/internet/nhhrc/publishing.nsf/Content/commission-1lp. Accessed 27 Oct 2014.

National Health Performance Authority. (2014). Time patients spent in emergency departments in 2012 and 2013. http://www.myhospitals.gov.au/Content/Reports/time-in-emergency-department/2014-05/pdf/MyHospitalsUpdate_TimeInEd_2012_13.pdf. Accessed 1 Sept 2014.

National Health Service (2014). Emergency and urgent care services. http://www.nhs.uk/NHSEngland/AboutNHSservices/Emergencyandurgentcareservices/Pages/AE.aspx. Accessed 1 Sept 2014.

National Public Health Partnership Secretariat (2000). *Public health practice in Australia today: A statement of core functions*. Melbourne: NPHPS.

Nitzan, U., Hirsch, E., Walter, G., Lurie, I., Aviram, S., & Bloch, Y. (2012). Comprehension and companionship in the emergency department as predictors of treatment adherence. *Australasian Psychiatry, 20*, 112–116.

NSW Clinical Excellence Commission (CEC) (2013). *Clinical incident management in the NSW public health system: July–December 2010*. Sydney: CEC.

NSW Department of Health. (2004). Clinical service redesign program: Redesigning a better patient journey, NSW Health, Sydney

NSW Department of Health. (2005). The New Patient Safety Program: Technical Paper, NSW Health, Sydney

NSW Health. (2012). *NSW Health Care Complaints Commission annual report 2011–12*. Sydney: NSW Health Care Complaints Commission.

Nugus, P., & Braithwaite, J. (2010). The dynamic interaction of quality and efficiency in the emergency department: Squaring the circle? *Social Science & Medicine, 70*, 511–517.

O'Gara, P., & Fairhurst, W. (2004). Therapeutic communication part 2: Strategies than can enhance the quality of the emergency care consultation. *Accident and Emergency Nursing, 12*, 201–207.

Olthuis G, Prns, C., Smits, M., van de Pas, H., Bierens. J., Baart, A. (2014). Matters of concern: A qualitative study of emergency care from the perspective of patients. *Annals of Emergency Medicine, 63*(1), 311–319.

Perez-Carceles, M., Gironda, J., Osuna, E., Falcon, M., & Luna, A. (2010). Is the right to information fulfilled in an emergency department? Patients' perceptions of the care provided. *Journal of Evaluation in Clinical Practice, 16*, 456–463.

Pham, J., Trueger, S., Hilton, J., Khare, R., Smith, J., Berstein, S. (2011). Interventions to improve patient centered care during times of emergency department overcrowding. *Academic Emergency Medicine, 18*, 1289–1294.

Redfern, E., Brown, R., & Vincent, C.A. (2009). Identifying vulnerabilities in communication in the emergency department: *Emergency Medicine Journal, 26*(9), 653–657.

Rhodes, K., Vieth, T., He, T., Miller, A., Howes, D., Bailey, O., Walter, J., Frankel, R., & Levinson, W. (2004). Resuscitating the physician–patient relationship: Emergency department communication in an academic medical center. *Annals of Emergency Medicine, 44*(3), 262–267.

Rider, E.A., Kurtz, S., Slade, D., Longmaid, H.E., Ho, M.-J., Pun, J.K.-H., Eggins, S., Branch, W.T. Jr. (2014). The international charter for human values in healthcare: An interprofessional global collaboration to enhance values and communication in healthcare. *Patient Education and Counseling, 96*(3), 273–280. doi:10.1016/j.pec.2014.06.017.

Samuels-Kalow, M., Stack, K., & Porter, S. (2011). Effective discharge communication in the emergency department. *Annals of Emergency Medicine, 60*, 152–159.

Slade, D., Scheeres, H., Manidis, M., Iedema, R., Dunston, R., Stein-Parbury, J., Matthiessen, C., Herke, M., & McGregor, J. (2008). Emergency communication: The discursive challenges facing emergency clinicians and patients in hospital emergency departments. *Discourse & Communication, 2*, 271–298. doi:10.1177/1750481308091910.

Slade, D., Manidis, M., McGregor, J., Scheeres, H., Stein-Parbury, J., Dunston, R., Stanton, N., Chandler, E., Matthiessen, C., & Herke, M. (2011). *Communicating in hospital emergency departments. Final report* (Vol 1). Sydney: University of Technology Sydney.

Sullivan, G. M., & Sargeant, J. (2011). Qualities of qualitative research: Part I. *Journal of Graduate Medical Education, 3*(4), 449–452.

Tam, A.Y.B., & Lau, F.L. (2000). A three-year review of complaints in emergency departments. *Hong Kong Journal of Emergency Medicine, 7*, 16–21.

UK Department of Health. (2000). An organisation with a memory. http://www.aagbi.org/sites/default/files/An%20organisation%20with%20a%20memory.pdf. Accessed 1 Sept 2014.

UK Department of Health. (2005). On the state of the public health: Annual report of the Chief Medical Officer. www.swpho.nhs.uk/resource/view.aspx?RID=30377. Accessed 1 Sept 2014.

US Institute of Medicine. (2001). Crossing the quality chasm: A new health system for the 21st century. National Academies Press.

US Joint Commission (2014). Sentinel event data: Root causes by event type 2004–2013. http://www.jointcommission.org/assets/1/18/Root_Causes_by_Event_Type_2004-2Q2013.pdf. Accessed 1 Sept 2014.

Vashi, A., & Rhodes, K. (2011). 'Sign right here and you're good to go': A content analysis of audiotaped emergency department discharge instructions. *Annals of Emergency Medicine, 57*(4), 315–322.

Vincent, C., Young, M., & Phillips, A. (1994). Why do people sue doctors? A study of patients and relatives taking legal action. *Lancet, 343*, 1609–1613.

Wilson, R. M., Runciman, W. B., Gibberd, R. W., Hamilton, J. D. (1995). The quality in Australian health care study. *Medical Journal of Australia, 458*(71), 163.

World Health Organization (WHO) (2007). Conceptual framework for the international classification for patient safety Version 1.0 for use in field testing.

Chapter 2
The Context of Communication in Emergency Departments

2.1 Introduction

The way we use language is always shaped by what we are communicating, and reflects the context in which we are doing so. The communicative challenges and risks in emergency departments arise directly from the unique contextual demands of the emergency department environment. In this chapter, we begin our account of communication demands of the emergency department by describing its characteristic features and seeing how these directly affect the nature of communication.

Patients experience many sites when they present to the emergency department—the waiting room, the ambulance bay, the triage, the acute and subacute sections and the 'bridge'. The bridge is the colloquial name given to the central communications hub in the emergency department of many hospitals in Australia.

Although it is referred to by other names, the bridge is a fixture in all emergency departments. Clinicians meet, talk, work on computers, often carry out the shift-to-shift handovers and write up the patient medical records in this central area. It is always full of action, with staff standing and sitting, moving into and out of the area. There are many communication and electronic artefacts (computer terminals, equipment), phones are constantly ringing and patient medical records are often scattered over the bench tops. The bridge is the communal centre of activity through which all clinicians move at some time during a shift. The purpose of the (usually) elevated platform that underpins the area and gives it its name is to provide a 'watchtower' view of the ambulance bay and resuscitation beds, and a good view of a number of the acute beds. It is also a central point for communication, both written and spoken.

We conducted a total of 1094 hrs of ethnographic observations in the different sections of emergency departments, which included shadowing key clinicians through parts of their shift, audio recording and taking detailed notes. These observations and shadowing yielded a rich graphic account of the activities, people, stories and interactions that take place daily in the triage room, the ambulance bay, the

© Springer-Verlag Berlin Heidelberg 2015
D. Slade et al., *Communicating in Hospital Emergency Departments*,
DOI 10.1007/978-3-662-46021-4_2

acute, subacute, emergency medicine unit (EMU), resuscitation areas, bridge and waiting room. Overall, they reveal a picture of busy, overstretched worksites with constant movement, talk and clinical action. This complexity is compounded for patients and carers who arrive as outsiders to the emergency department environment.

To set the scene, we begin our description of the emergency department context by presenting a vignette of a day during which we shadowed a senior nurse manager in one large metropolitan emergency department. We followed the nurse throughout her shift on a Monday following a typically busy weekend. Several patients who had arrived over the weekend were still awaiting admission to a hospital ward. Others were waiting to be seen by specialists from other areas of the hospital, unable to be discharged from the emergency department until they were cleared. The description is based on the observation notes and audio recordings of the nurse's interactions. It clearly demonstrates the high stress and intense demands of working in emergency departments, and the significant challenges faced by clinicians in them.

We then describe the various contextual factors that characterise emergency departments and make them unique, and demonstrate how these contextual factors manifest in specific communication practices in emergency department care.

2.2   Setting the Scene: A Busy Day in an Emergency Department

It was a bad weekend. The director of the emergency department (ED) had been called on Sunday at 2 am and informed that the situation in the ED was critical. Now Monday, 1.45 pm, it is still critical. The primary problems are bed space and acuity. Patients are spilling into the corridors and out of the exits. A senior nurse working in the ED complains that staff cannot even see the patients—there are just too many of them, piled up and out of view. At around 1:50 pm 'another' level 3 page goes out, notifying the hospital that the ED is in a situation of overcrowding and in need of the wider hospital's support. Already over the ambulance threshold (with seven patients waiting in the bay), ambulance officers have begun to queue around the entry to the department.

A bed manager comes down to allocate beds among the waiting patients but gets nowhere. The access to beds is not there, creating further queues. The queue for beds at 2 pm is nine people long. A senior doctor suggests that they start doing the rounds to find people who are better and 'to see who we can get rid of'. The senior nurse on duty replies that there is no-one who can be moved. A young girl has been in an ED bed since the night before. The orthopaedic ward refuses to take her until her neck is formally cleared and documented. The orthopaedic registrar had been on his way down to do this but has been called away to do something else.

Two staff specialists are 'trapped' in the ambulance bay. Although this is a non-treatment area they have started treating patients anyway, taking patient bloods, getting ECGs. With every patient there is an ambulance officer—sitting around, waiting to handover his or her patient when a bed becomes available. They monitor their patients, although regulations prevent them from administering any care. Mostly, they just have to 'sit there' and wait. Another ambulance turns up making the queue ten patients long.

A senior nurse goes to call the hospital bed managers but is informed that all bed managers are unable to come down as 'they're in meetings'. She calls them anyway, informing them that it 'is critically unsafe down here'. The researchers are told that those words 'critically unsafe' get a response. The senior doctor and nurse try to work out whether they can send any of the patients down to EMU to free up a bed. They agree that five can go; however, in the end they only manage to free up one bed. Another ambulance arrives. There are now 11 patients in the ambulance bay and the ED now 'does not have resusc capacity'[1]. Non-resusc patients are occupying the beds dedicated to this level of care. The senior nurse, still having received no response from the bed managers, writes to the program executive, pleading for managerial staff to support them.

A further admission is declared by one of the doctors in the ambulance bay. A senior nurse does a round of the ambulance bay getting briefed on the waiting list—several patients have been sitting in this area since 10 am. It is now almost 2 pm. No-one has been treated. Meanwhile, the ambulances have begun to queue behind the doors at the entry to the ED. The doctors have 'no visual line' to those patients. One of these patients is diagnosed as critically unwell with a pericardial effusion. It needs to be tapped urgently. Another patient has a severe allergic reaction. Another has had a severe epileptic seizure. A 'psych' patient occupying one of the beds is asked to move into a seat to make space for the patient with the allergic reaction. Another mental health patient, who has been in the ED for an inordinate number of hours without a bed, is moved into the corridor. Meanwhile, the patient with the allergic reaction still goes untreated—it is predicted that she will lose an airway if she is not addressed shortly.

The senior nurse walks to the EMU and finds there are five beds there. She decides to override the department's own policies and assigns five non-urgent patients' beds down there. Instantly, the ED beds that were freed up are filled again. It is now 2.20 pm and there are still six people waiting in the ambulance bay. The girl waiting for the orthopaedic registrar has still not been moved and there has been no sign of the bed managers. A nurse explains to the researchers that three beds in the ED are being blocked because the patients cannot be transferred into wards. One of these patients is a 98-year-old woman who has been in the ED since 2 pm the day before—she cannot be moved because there is simply no bed for her to go to. Staff attempt to clear

---

[1] 'Resusc' refers to a reserved bed where patients who need resuscitation can be put.

the beds in 'resusc' so that they can regain resusc capacity. Every patient they approach is waiting for a bed to be freed in a ward. None can be moved. There are no clinical beds and no mental health beds in the hospital. Further, despite three mental health admissions, only one 'special' nurse has been provided—they have been given one-third of what is required for safety.

Two beds become free in EMU and resusc capacity is temporarily regained. The acting director of nursing comes down to sort out the ward blocks. Just as the staff begin to regain control, the computer board refreshes itself and sends out the message that the ED can take two more patients. This is anything but the case. A new patient who has arrived is suspected of having Legionella and needs to be isolated. Seconds later a mental health patient arrives without a 'special' nurse in attendance. Staff attempt contact with the Mental Health Unit to clarify whether they have beds. At 3 pm, the second bed manager comes down. Moments later the orthopaedic registrar arrives to make a decision about the girl's neck. He clears the spine immediately and the girl is moved. Doctors remain in the ambulance bay, attempting to provide whatever care possible to those patients not yet able to be placed in a clinical area in the ED. A nurse comments to the researchers: 'This is where it gets unsafe. Doctors in the ambulance bay with trolleys and with needles. All you need is a psychotic patient in there to go off and all hell will break loose.'

The senior nurse does another round of the bay and finds a 'potential SBE'[2] in need of urgent antibiotic treatment. She also meets a man with myocardial infarction who has had his ECG delayed. He needs to go on a bed immediately. Meanwhile, the patient suspected of having Legionella has still not been isolated. As predicted by ED staff, the man with infarction has an abnormal reading on his ECG and is an admission. Behind him, staff frantically make phone calls trying to free up beds and create movement for patient flow. The ambulance bay is still spilling with patients and trolleys and it is virtually impossible to walk freely around the department. A senior nurse asks the ambulance officers to attempt to make a clear way. Finally a man with hypoglycaemia who arrived at 11.30 am is offloaded from the ambulance bay onto a bed at 3.15 pm.

There is a woman in the corridor waiting on a trolley and obstructing the path to resusc. One staff member, on seeing her, groans: 'If they have a cardiac now, how do they run through there?' She is moved onto a seat in the main area so that she can be watched by staff. Minutes later the radio announces that a cardiac arrest is on its way in. There is no bed empty in the resuscitation rooms but staff manage to clear an empty space in one by putting all occupied beds in the one resuscitation room. One of the patients in Resuscitation 2 has been there all day. Around six minutes after being announced, the cardiac arrest arrives and is rushed into resusc. Her heart stops beating; they 'call it'—

---

[2] SBE: Shortness of breath on exertion.

they are not able to bring her back. The senior doctor and the social worker go to see the family of the cardiac patient, who have been waiting in a nearby room, to explain that the patient has died.

Meanwhile, outside, the patient who had an epileptic seizure still sits in the ambulance bay waiting for treatment. The staff believe he will have another seizure soon. Nine more patients are about to arrive at the ED by ambulance. There is still nowhere to offload them. Waiting to be seen are a young man with a dislocated shoulder with pain at 8/10 and 'a febrile old lady'. A nurse re-categorises them as Category 2 'so someone can just start seeing them'. It is decided that at least two patients who have been in the department all day will be held overnight—there are no beds to accommodate them …

This scene clearly demonstrates that when presentations are relentless the situation reaches a critical point. Comments made by staff highlighted the lack of resources and inadequate staffing in the emergency departments, presenting a work environment that is cumulatively and increasingly challenging.

2.3   The Context of the Emergency Department

Emergency departments are sites of significant and increasing contextual complexity. This complexity stems from a number of factors, including operational hours and uncapped patient loads; the increased demand for emergency department care; the short term and an episodic nature of emergency department care and the impact it has on clinician–patient relationships; the multidisciplinary nature of emergency department healthcare teams; the tertiary function of emergency departments as a practical training facilities for student and junior doctors and nurses; their linguistic and cultural diversity; and, finally, their reliance on spoken language as the main medium of communication between clinicians, and between clinicians and patients.

2.3.1   Operational Hours and Uncapped Patient Loads

Emergency departments operate 24 hrs a day, 7 days a week. At any time, patients suffering a range of acute illnesses and injuries can arrive at the emergency department door. As such, while emergency medicine may be described as a specialty in its own right, the range of patient injuries and illnesses that emergency department clinicians must diagnose and treat means that it can also be described as 'encompassing every specialty that exists in the world of medicine' (registrar, hospital B).

There are no limits to the number of patient presentations—rather, emergency departments have uncapped patient loads. As one senior doctor we interviewed explained, unlike 'a ward [in which I can say] we've got 30 beds and that's it, we can't take anymore … it doesn't matter whether we're prepared or not, we have to be prepared and we have to provide that service. We're a service that has excess demands all the time for the resources available' (medical specialist, hospital A).

One flow-on effect of the combination of the operational hours and uncapped demand is that emergency departments must be staffed by changing shifts of clinicians. As a result, patients are likely to be cared for by many different doctors and nurses during their time in the emergency department. In turn, emergency clinicians will care for patients simultaneously (Redfern et al. 2009, p. 653) as they balance the organisational and policy requirements of providing care to all patients who arrive at the emergency department, within specified time frames.

2.3.2   Increased Presentations and Overcrowding in Emergency Departments

The demand for emergency care is on the rise around the world (see, e.g. Committee on the Future of Emergency Care in the United States Health System 2006, pp. 38–39; Lowthian et al. 2012). In Australia, emergency department presentations have risen on a steady incline for the last 5 years. Between 2008 and 2013, presentations increased by an average of 2.9 % per year (Australian Institute of Health and Welfare 2013, p. 7). The peak times for patient arrival tend to be during the weekends and on Mondays, between the hours of 10 am and 12 noon (Australian Institute of Health and Welfare 2013, p. 12).

Emergency departments around the world need to have a process for determining the priority of patient treatments based on the severity of the patient's condition. This process, referred to as 'triage', is essential if resources are such that not everyone can be treated as soon as they arrive. The triage categories vary from country to country—in Australia, the triage categories are on a scale of 1–5 (referred to as the Australasian Triage Scale (ATS). The scale has been in use since 1994. The scale consists of 5 levels, with 1 being the most critical (resuscitation), and 5 being the least critical (nonurgent). In order of urgency and priority, these categories are resuscitation, emergency, urgent, semi-urgent and nonurgent (Table 2.1).

Nationally, most patient presentations fall into the latter three categories (Australian Institute of Health and Welfare 2013, p. 17). The increasing use of emergency departments by nonurgent patients is a worldwide phenomenon, and reflects many

Table 2.1 Australasian Triage Scale

Triage level	Description	Should be seen by provider within (min)
1	Resuscitation	0
2	Emergency	10
3	Urgent	30
4	Semi-urgent	60
5	Nonurgent	120

factors, including the 24 hrs accessibility and availability of emergency department care, patient's desire to avoid prolonged waiting times for appointments in primary healthcare contexts, perceptions of emergency departments as one-stop healthcare sites for multiple tests and access to a range of specialisations and rising costs of healthcare in private settings (Durand et al. 2012; Committee on the Future of Emergency Care in the United States Health System 2006, pp. 38–39).

This increased demand for nonurgent care in the emergency department setting results in many patients experiencing extensive waiting time before being admitted. They are often unaware of the rationale behind triage, and are subsequently frustrated by the delay between their initial arrival at the emergency department and receiving treatment. The often unmanageable demand also increases the risks to patient safety inherent in the triage system. For example, many clinicians reported the limitations of this practice, citing lack of clinical expertise by the clinicians responsible for triage which can result in under-triaging (so underestimating critical nature of presenting condition), not considering differences in injury severities and survival probabilities between types of trauma, and not taking age into account (see Navin and Sacco 2010).

The increased number of presentations are associated with overcrowding, with widespread reports of overcrowding in emergency departments around the world raising doubts about the capacity of emergency services to provide safe care (Lowthian et al. 2012). There is increasing evidence that overcrowding affects patient safety. Bernstein et al. 2009, p. 1 state that:

> A growing body of data suggests that ED crowding is associated both with objective clinical endpoints, such as mortality, as well as clinically important processes of care, such as time to treatment for patients with time-sensitive conditions such as pneumonia. At least two domains of quality of care, safety and timeliness, are compromised by ED crowding.

On 31 August 2014, hospital D's emergency department clinical director said on the online edition of the daily *ABC news* that he was very concerned about the increased patient presentation numbers to the emergency department and that 'current patient numbers are unsafe and unsustainable'.

He said that the presentations to the emergency department have increased by 7%, and that overcrowding not only affects the patient experience but more critically their safety:

> Once you've been seen and you have a diagnosis, how long you stay in emergency and how crowded emergency is has impacts on health. It increases time in hospital, it increases costs, it increases complications and in fact it increases mortality.(Dr Michael Hall, emergency department clinical director, online Australian Broadcast Commission news, 31 August 2014)

The continuing rise in patient presentations presents significant challenges to both the quality and safety of the patient experience, with significant evidence from around the world that the risk of adverse events is increasing due to overcrowding (Schull et al. 2002).

2.3.3 Short-term, Episodic Patient Care: The Lack of Familiarity Between Emergency Department Patients and Clinicians

Emergency departments are set up to provide short-term, episodic, urgent and life-saving care. The primary objectives of emergency department care are to determine as efficiently as possible a patient's diagnosis, and to decide whether the patient can be treated within the emergency department and discharged, or whether they need to be admitted to the wider hospital or referred elsewhere for ongoing care and supervision. The challenge for emergency department clinicians is to make these determinations in the absence of any readily accessible medical records, known medical histories or established relationships with patients. In the words of one staff specialist we interviewed 'Our patients are unknown, they're new, so they don't come in with the diagnosis tattooed on their forehead and that is often very difficult for people who don't work in emergency to understand' (staff specialist, hospital A). Although some patients may return to the emergency department for follow-up care, for most, their relationships with their emergency department clinicians will cease following their discharge from the emergency department. As a result, it is imperative for patient safety that patients leave the emergency department with a clear understanding of their diagnosis and their clinician's recommended treatment regimen postdischarge. Without this, as Perez-Carceles et al. (2010, p. 456) note, compliance with discharge instructions will be unlikely, as there will be no subsequent contact between clinicians and patients, and therefore no further opportunity for patients to clarify their understanding, or clinicians to ensure patient comprehension.

2.3.4 The Physical Environment: Noise Levels, Privacy and Comfort

A flow-on effect of the short-term, functional nature of emergency department care is that they are not designed for prolonged patient stays. As one clinician commented, the emergency department is 'a terrible environment for people to sit in for 24 hrs, there's no doubt about that. Our beds aren't designed for people to stay, we don't have enough showers, we don't—we're not meant to be that' (senior staff specialist). Researcher observations of the physical environment of each emergency department we studied paint the picture of crowded, cold, sterile and clinical spaces, summarised in Table 2.2.

Emergency departments are also notoriously noisy clinical environments, filled with the constant sounds of medical equipment, patient monitors, computers, overhead announcements, phone calls and conversations between patients and clinicians and amongst clinicians themselves. As Short et al. (2011, pp. 28–29) found, the highest noise levels tend to be in the resuscitation areas and acute sections of the emergency department, often exceeding established recommendations of sound levels for patient areas and wards. Exposure to high levels of constant noise in clinical settings has been correlated with increased agitation and psychological distress, patient confusion, staff exhaustion and medical and nursing errors (Short et al. 2011).

Table 2.2 Layout and space in the five emergency departments studied

Hospital A	Hospital B	Hospital C	Hospital D	Hospital E
Crowded; cluttered walls; white; bright; few windows; cubicles defined by curtains	Beige; brown; clinical; ordered; windows; clean walls; cubicles defined by curtains	Windowless; ordered; antiseptic; bright yellow; cubicles defined by curtains	Has some windows; bright; antiseptic; cubicles defined by curtains	Windows in one part of acute; none in subacute or EMU; walls are green; cubicles defined by curtains

In our research, we found that the level of noise in the emergency departments frequently affected the audibility of patient–staff interactions, with clinicians and patients regularly needing to repeat themselves in order to hear one another. Further, as patient beds were often only separated from each other by curtains, this provided very little privacy for their occupants. Throughout our research we observed that often patient–clinician conversations were clearly audible from the next-door beds. As one intern (hospital A) said to us:

> I often think … yeah I don't … I think I would have to be seriously ill to go to an ED (laughter) just because I think it would be such a frustrating experience and particularly late at night because it never closes down … the lights are always on, there's always noise and there's always people and I think if I felt like that person probably feels, the last thing I would want would be a big noisy room with people running around and no one coming when I press my button and… so that sort of thing. So I think it's a very frustrating and prolonged experience for them. I think once they're on the wards it's a little bit … far more sane 'cause it's a little bit more settled.

2.3.5 Multidisciplinary Healthcare Teams

Emergency department healthcare teams are made up of doctors, nurses and allied health professionals (although the major disciplinary divisions are between doctors and nurses). All have different roles and priorities in the management and treatment of patients who present to the emergency department. Nurses will typically manage the ongoing care of patients in the emergency department (e.g. administer pain relief, monitor each patient's stability and comfort), while doctors will diagnose, establish a treatment plan and determine whether a patient can be discharged from the emergency department or admitted to a hospital ward for further observation and care. Notably, while the disciplines work side by side, in all but one of the emergency departments we researched, there was very little evidence of interdisciplinary collaboration throughout patient journeys. Rather, we observed clinicians attending patients' bedsides individually and asynchronously, undertaking discipline-specific tasks and care. We also frequently observed tensions between doctors and nurses relating to the performance of tasks that traversed traditional disciplinary boundaries. The lack of interdisciplinary practice also led to a lack of familiarity between staff of different disciplines:

Junior doctor: Do you do lines?
Nurse: Not on him, he's got terrible veins. Technically it's your job doctor.
Junior doctor: I know.
Nurse: I don't do lines, because I'm very good at blowing them.

And in another emergency department:

Junior doctor: Are you looking after the patient in bed 10?
Nurse: I'm a float nurse.
Junior doctor: Is that a 'yes' or a 'no'?
Nurse: That's a 'no'.

In the following sections, we discuss that the multidisciplinary nature of emergency department care will often translate to different communicative roles being undertaken by nurses and doctors in their interactions with patients. It also produces complex networks of care that surround each patient's journey in the emergency department.

2.3.6   Joint Role of Emergency Departments as Training Facilities

In Australia, as elsewhere, emergency departments are training grounds for junior doctors and nurses. As the final report of the Special Commission of Enquiry into Acute Care Services in NSW Public Hospitals pointed out, most of the acute care services for noncritical patients are performed by junior doctors (interns, residents, registrars, career medical officers and locums). In essence the report notes, Australian acute health services are training grounds for junior doctors. (Garling 2008, p. 428).

Junior clinicians with varying levels of experience and expertise learn on the job and predominantly focus on the immediate clinical task in front of them. A central component of the work of senior clinicians is supervising and guiding their junior colleagues. In all emergency departments we researched, however, senior clinicians (both nurses and doctors) were far less in number than their junior counterparts, which stretched the capacity of senior staff to perform their supervisory roles. As a director of one emergency department explained in reference to the medical discipline: 'Junior medical staff ... they're learning so ... they're going to make mistakes ... And we are understaffed with consultants here. So [as a senior doctor] when you're on the floor you've got everybody coming at you all the time for 10 hours looking for direction'. Indeed, across our interviews, nearly all senior clinicians described the key challenge of their work as stemming from the constant interruptions they faced as they multitasked their competing responsibilities of supervising junior colleagues, performing direct clinical care and facilitating patient flow across the department. This was particularly emphasised by senior medical staff members who bear the primary responsibility not only for individual patient diagnosis and disposition decisions, but also for negotiating the transfer of patients from the emergency department to other hospital wards. As one senior staff specialist explained:

The ability to function … is impaired dramatically by the constant interruptions that happen and that's not a criticism of anybody it's just the way that we work. I tracked it one shift and you know, one shift—I think I answered the 'phone 20 times, I saw eight of my own patients, I reviewed 20 of the interns' (junior) patients in person and discussed another 15 or 20. If you sort of divide 60 or 70 little work tasks into an eight or ten-hour day you realise that's why you never get to concentrate. And that's very difficult—to concentrate on one, to force yourself to concentrate on one thing when there are other things going on.

This tertiary teaching function of emergency departments, although not often explained to patients, plays out throughout the patient's journey, and becomes particularly visible through the order in which patients, triaged in the less urgent categories of 3–5, will encounter and interact with junior and senior doctors. As will be discussed further in Chap. 3, junior doctors will generally be the ones who carry out the emergency department patient's first medical consultation. They will take the patient's history and explore their condition, then formulate their test plans and an initial diagnosis. The junior doctor will then consult with a senior doctor who, as noted above, has overall responsibility for the patient's ultimate diagnosis and disposition.

Depending on the complexity of the patient's presentation, the senior doctor may then conduct another consultation with the patient, either with or without the junior doctor, to confirm the junior doctor's initial assessment. What this means for the patient is that they will often encounter at least two doctors over the course of their emergency department care, with varying levels of expertise and experience. Further, as senior doctors double-check the clinical assessments of their junior colleagues, patients will frequently find themselves being asked the same questions over and over again, without being aware why this is happening.

2.3.7   Time Constraints

Emergency department staff and patients are constrained by time in far more extreme ways than in other professional or private contexts. Few emergency department participants (clinicians and patients) have any real control over their own time and the time taken for medical analyses. Staff members are pressured to move, talk and think quickly, while patients can spend long periods in holding patterns, waiting on results, diagnoses, X-rays and returning staff. Since we conducted this research, the Australian Federal Government has introduced a National Emergency Access Target ('NEAT') which requires most patients to be diagnosed, treated and discharged from Australian emergency departments within 4 h. Modelled on the UK's National Health Service Plan, the target was driven by research and state government inquiries linking prolonged waiting times with poor patient health outcomes (Crawford et al. 2013, pp. 2–3). To date, there has been little research which has investigated the impact of NEAT on the overall quality of emergency patient care in Australia. It remains to be seen whether its introduction has indeed improved patient outcomes, or whether the added time pressure on staff to process patients through emergency departments has compromised the interpersonal dimensions of emergency care and other benchmarks of quality healthcare practice (Crawford et al. 2013).

2.3.8   Face-to-Face Spoken Communication

Face-to-face spoken communication dominates emergency department work. Indeed, emergency medicine can be characterised as a predominantly spoken discipline (Coiera et al. 2002, p. 417; Spencer et al. 2004; Woloshynowych et al. 2007; Kee et al. 2012, p. 297). Clinicians will talk to patients, to each other, to hospital staff and to clinicians and health workers in the broader healthcare community, with written records playing a secondary role. In the previous observational studies of emergency department, clinicians' work have shown that clinicians will engage in between 36 and 49 communication events per hour (Coiera et al. 2002, p. 416). As described above, the communication loads for clinicians will often increase according to higher levels of seniority (see also Fairbanks et al. 2007, p. 403), and be characterised by interruptions and multitasking. Indeed, one senior doctor we interviewed estimated that over the course of his shift, he would speak to at least 100 different people:

> I will talk to patients, I talk to patients' families, I would talk to all the other members of staff, both nursing and medical staff and also the various Allied Health staff such as physiotherapists. I would talk to the diagnostic support infrastructure such as having negotiations with the pathology department, the X-ray department. I would talk to the ambulance staff. I would talk to the clerical staff and I would talk to representatives of the in-patient teams. And many days I have gripes about various things and I talk to the administration as well. So I would talk to quite possibly 100 given people in a day. (Staff specialist)

Every one of these spoken interactions can potentially involve a misunderstanding, a subtle change of meaning or interpretation, and as that information then gets passed onto someone else, the chance of changed nuances or of information omitted or forgotten is very high. This is particularly the case in clinical handover where often crucial patient information is not picked up on, not written in their medical records or inaccurate (see Eggins and Slade 2012; Eggins and Slade forthcoming). Pressures of time and tradition also mean that a lot of what is spoken is not recorded in the patient's written records, although there is a growing policy emphasis on improving written healthcare communication in these settings. As you will see in Figs. 2.1, 2.2, 2.3 and 2.4 below, spoken communication load for emergency department patients also tends to be exceptionally high. They must communicate the nature of their symptoms and their histories within a relatively short period of time and to a multitude of staff, and comprehend complex information provided by many different clinicians.

2.3.9   Linguistic and Cultural Diversity

Most countries around the world are characterised by an increasingly multicultural population. This is reflected in the cultural and linguistic diversity of emergency department patients and of clinicians—many of whom have been trained overseas. This linguistic diversity introduces other dimensions to the spoken communication loads experienced by emergency department participants—with family members or (less often) trained interpreters acting as cross-cultural and language mediators between patients and hospital staff, and clinicians needing to be culturally sensitive and appropriate both with other colleagues and with patients.

All of the factors outlined above make emergency departments unique healthcare contexts. Individuals and teams with very different disciplinary, cultural and experiential backgrounds are expected to somehow work together in a coherent and systematic way in a high-paced, stressful and unpredictable environment. This complexity does not mean that the emergency departments are chaotic. On the contrary, we found that the patient trajectory is complex but highly systematised, although systems are not made transparent to the public or to patients. The characteristics listed in the Sects. (2.3.1–2.3.9) do, however, result in communicative complexity, reflected in intricate networks of care for each patient, high communication burdens for patients and clinicians, and competing agendas between clinicians, patients and the organisation, all of which can significantly affect the quality and safety of the patient experience.

2.4   The Communicative Complexity of the Emergency Department

In this section, we illustrate how contextual factors are reflected in emergency department communication practices.

2.4.1   Networks of Care

As described above, emergency departments are multidisciplinary and cross-level (senior–junior) healthcare sites. As a result, emergency department patients will encounter and communicate with many different doctors, nurses, allied health workers and administrative personnel throughout their care. On average, we observed that between 8 and 15 staff were involved in the care of each patient we recorded. Each of these transitions is vulnerable to miscommunication and to lost or changed information. The clinical handovers between clinicians were mainly spoken (and so details can easily be forgotten or misremembered), and interdisciplinary handovers were rare. To illustrate the complex networks of care that arise, we present the experiences of two patients.

2.4.1.1   Denton's Case

The first patient consultation we described is with Denton[3]. Denton was an 80-year-old man who presented to the emergency department with shortness of breath and a fever. He spent five and a half hours in the emergency department from triage to

---

[3] All patient names throughout this book are pseudonyms.

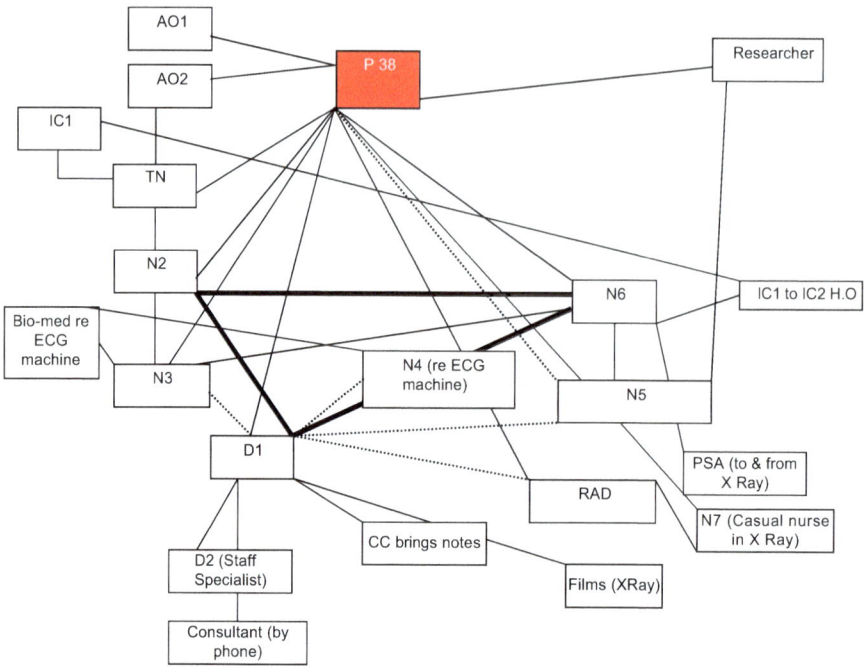

Fig. 2.1 Network of care for Denton (Manidis et al. 2009; Slade et al. 2011)

admission. Over the course of his care, Denton interacted directly with two ambulance officers, 10 nurses, two doctors, one radiographer, one orderly, one communication clerk and one researcher. In the background, at least five other emergency department staff members were involved in his care, although they did not directly communicate with him or approach his bedside. Figure 2.1 shows the network of care that encompassed Denton's time in the emergency department. It represents those who approached his bedside during his stay.

During his 125 min of recorded interactions (this is the time out of a total five and a half hour stay in the emergency department that Denton was with clinicians), Denton had 243 communicative encounters with clinicians. 'Encounter diagrams' document the interaction. They clearly demonstrate the communicative complexity for both patients and clinicians in emergency departments, as in each of these encounters there is a possibility of a communication misunderstanding or breakdown. Figure 2.2 captures these interactions in sequence, with a square marking every time someone spoke to him or about him at the bedside.

The encounters were coded based on detailed field notes and the transcripts. The manner of coding followed that of Manidis (2013):

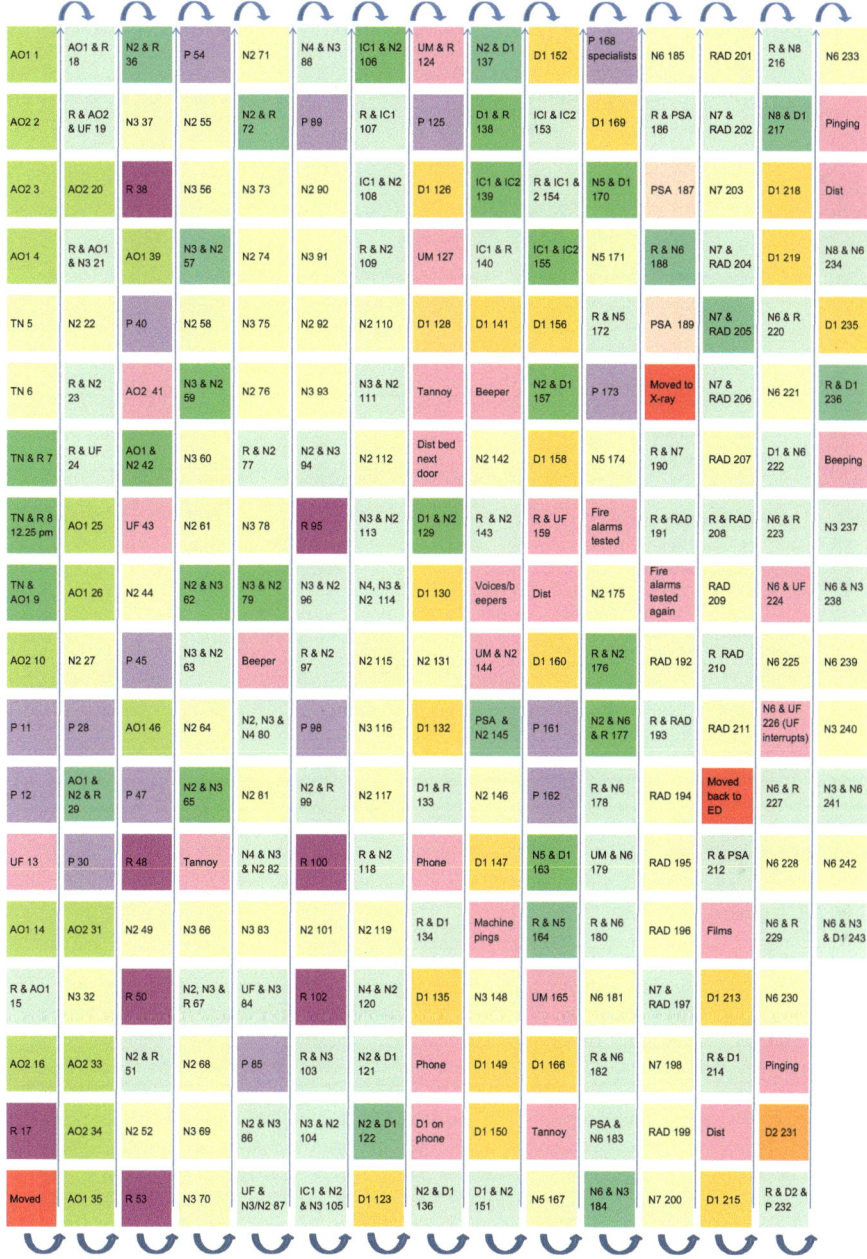

a

Fig. 2.2 Sequence of interactions with and around Denton

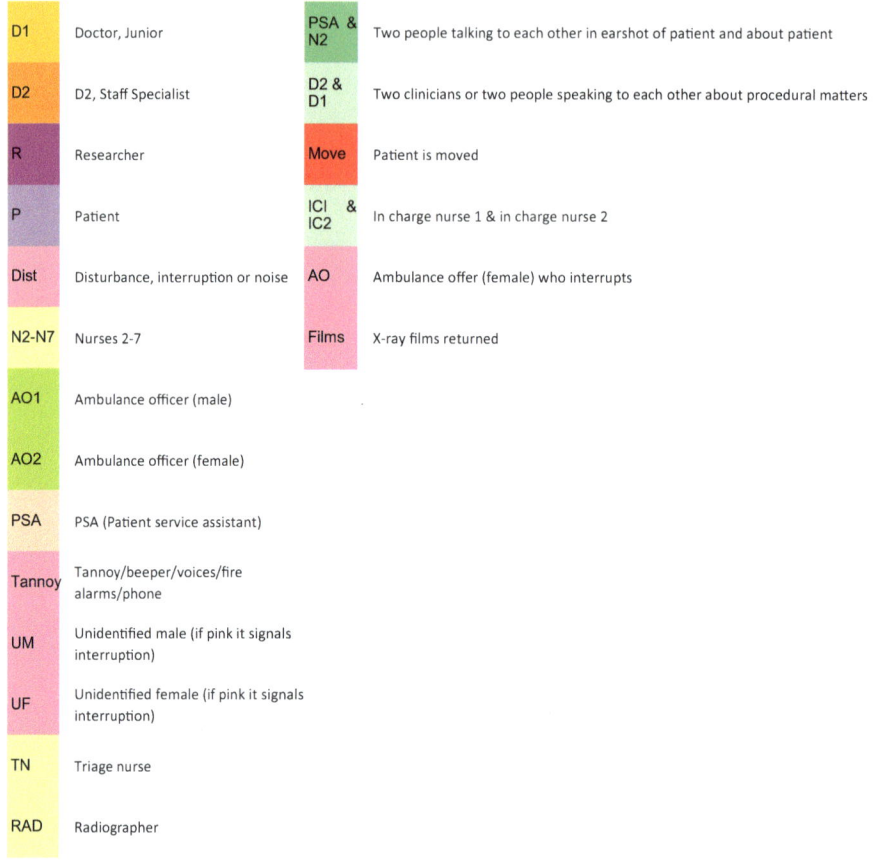

D1	Doctor, Junior	PSA & N2	Two people talking to each other in earshot of patient and about patient
D2	D2, Staff Specialist	D2 & D1	Two clinicians or two people speaking to each other about procedural matters
R	Researcher	Move	Patient is moved
P	Patient	ICI & IC2	In charge nurse 1 & in charge nurse 2
Dist	Disturbance, interruption or noise	AO	Ambulance offer (female) who interrupts
N2-N7	Nurses 2-7	Films	X-ray films returned
AO1	Ambulance officer (male)		
AO2	Ambulance officer (female)		
PSA	PSA (Patient service assistant)		
Tannoy	Tannoy/beeper/voices/fire alarms/phone		
UM	Unidentified male (if pink it signals interruption)		
UF	Unidentified female (if pink it signals interruption)		
TN	Triage nurse		
RAD	Radiographer		

b

Fig. 2.2 (continued)

I coded each new action and/or each new interlocutor with a patient on the transcript. I coded patient relocations in the ED, each noise disturbance or interruption (by tea ladies, for example)… I identify each of these encounters, particularly each nurse's and doctor's saying and/or doing (action) as episodic, what Schatzki calls an 'event' (Schatzki 2011), a bounded physical or discursive action … The colour codings indicate different interlocutors (the processes), for example, when nurses and doctors re-introduce themselves or re-question the patient after an absence etc. They also indicate the content (i. e. whether nurses and doctors are talking about the patient or about their work). The colour codings also indicate when the patient speaks up, makes a request, or exercises their agency. (Manidis 2013, pp. 77–78)

As shown in Fig. 2.1, during the entire consultation Denton experienced 225 encounters, which were recorded in 2 hrs of dialogue with doctors and nurses and a radiographer. This means that Denton engaged with someone, or his consultation was interrupted by someone or something, every 32 secs. Denton was moved three times; saw one doctor, one radiographer and seven nurses. Nurse 3 returned to the bedside 20 times and nurse 2 a total of 18 times to engage with the patient.

Denton's consultations were difficult for the doctors and nurses as he was very sick. There were 18 interruptions to the consultation by others, mostly to do with the management of the care of other patients. At encounter 168, two-third of the way through the consultation, Denton asked 'Who are my specialists?', indicating his confusion about his care experience.

By that stage three ambulance officers, seven nurses, two doctors, one triage nurse and one researcher, all had multiple conversations with or about him at close proximity. Additionally, two team leaders in charge, two unidentified male voices, two phone calls the doctor had taken and several overhead announcements had occurred around him. Denton had also been moved once.

Some evident tensions between the junior doctor and the nurses, the broken equipment and testing the fire alarms all would have contributed to the overall confusion of Denton's experience. Denton's desire to make sense of his care regime suggests room for practice improvements around the structuring of discursive and clinical practices across and even within disciplinary boundaries by doctors and nurses at emergency department bedsides.

2.4.1.2   Dulcie's Case

The second consultation illustrating the communicative complexity of emergency department consultations is that of Dulcie, a 63-year-old woman. When she arrived at the emergency department, with a letter from her general practitioner (GP), she was very ill. Dulcie was having trouble breathing and was triaged immediately. There was no bed available but the triage nurse began treatment by organising for one of the ambulance officers, who was undertaking extended care training, to take blood to get a reading of her blood gases. This can be a very painful procedure if not conducted properly, and as Dulcie was sitting in a chair in the ambulance she felt a lot of discomfort. She was moved after a while into a bed in the isolation room as there were no other beds available.

Dulcie had 326 encounters (see Figs. 2.3 and 2.4 below) involving three doctors, seven nurses, three ambulance officers, one clerical staff member, one tea lady, one researcher, an orderly and a radiographer. There were four other people who engaged with her in the bedside space, but who are unidentified. See Fig. 2.3 below for the network of care around Dulcie.

Dulcie spent 8 hrs in the emergency department before being admitted. We recorded her interactions over a period of 2 hrs and 16 min, which means she had an encounter every 25 secs. Dulcie initiated many of the encounters herself—a total of 101 in all.

Figure 2.4 shows the encounters that Dulcie had. The sheer number of encounters over the 4 hrs period as well as the environmental and contextual dynamics of the consultation are immediately visible.

Dulcie was a trained assistant in nursing, and said she had learnt that one needed to ask in order to find out what was happening: 'I do [ask a lot of questions], 'cause I've—with the course [AIN], I mean, if you don't ask you don't get—well they can either tell you to shut up == or ( )'.

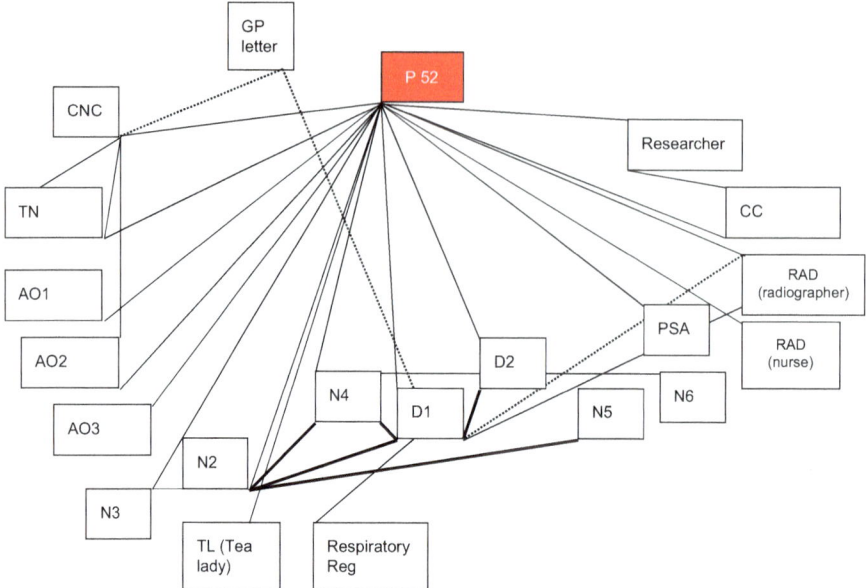

Fig. 2.3 Network of care for Dulcie (after Manidis et al. 2009; Slade et al. 2011)

The consultations that Dulcie had with the different clinicians was notable for its training component, involving three novice practitioners: a junior doctor, a new 'grad' nurse and an ambulance officer who was undertaking the practical component of an extended care paramedic's course. The senior doctor closely supervised the junior doctor. The junior doctor was very attentive throughout, gave lots of explanations and developed a good rapport with the patient, but did admit at one point that he was getting Dulcie mixed up with another of his patients who also had a lung condition. The junior doctor reconnected 24 times with Dulcie in new or time-separated encounters. He was unable to insert the cannula, a task then undertaken by the senior doctor. The ambulance officer *'was doing what we call ECP at the moment which is Extended Care Paramedics'* program and took the blood gas reading in the beginning from Dulcie. Nurse 2 was a new graduate and also worked closely under the supervision of nurse 4. Nurse 2 reinitiated an encounter with Dulcie 14 separate times and nurse 4 a total of 16 times.

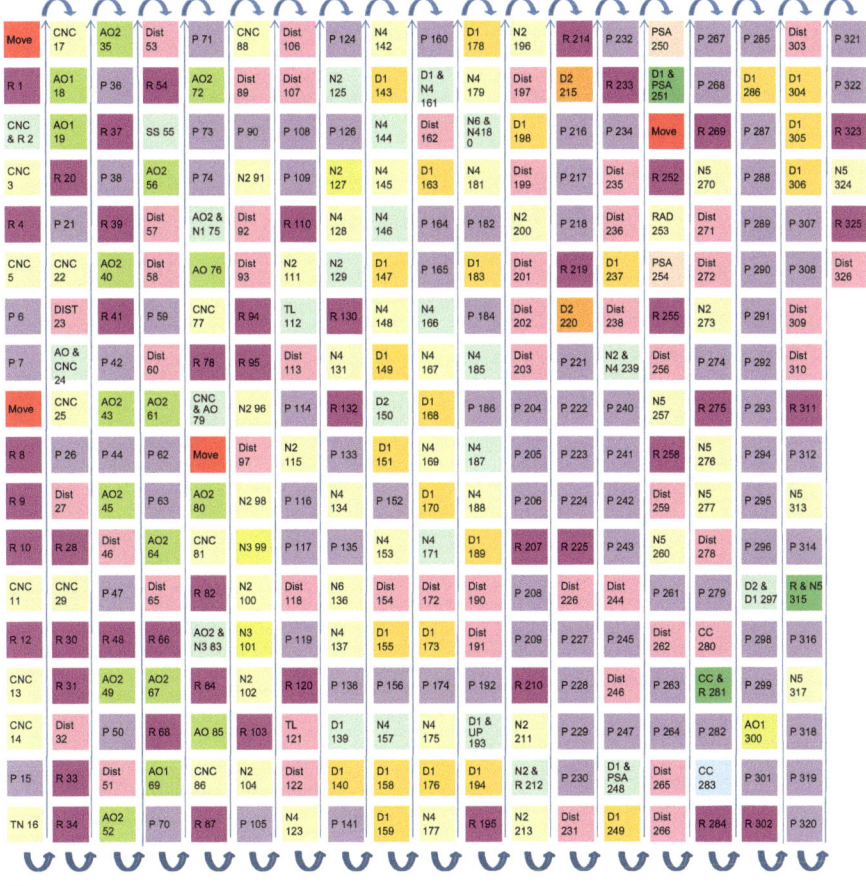

a

Fig. 2.4   Encounters for Dulcie (after Manidis et al. 2009; Slade et al. 2011)

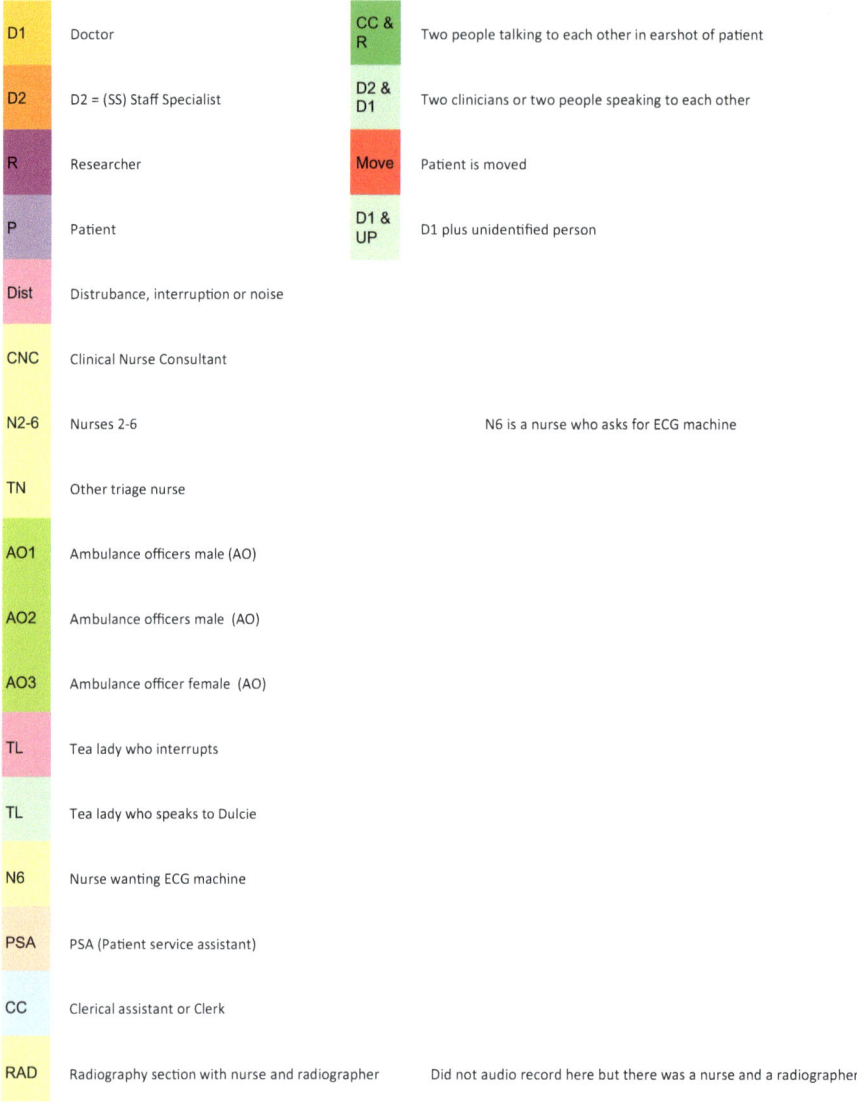

b

Fig. 2.4 (continued)

2.4.2 Risks to Knowledge/Information Transfer

As Dulcie's example suggests, with so many different people involved in each patient's care, there are real risks that knowledge and information about patients will be lost in the complex care network. In the words of one communication clerk at one emergency department, the everyday reality of managing knowledge about patients (in this case patient notes) is a time consuming task:

Researcher: Do you spend any time looking for patient notes?
Clerk: Probably more than anybody else.
Researcher: How much time? [Laughter]
Clerk: I would probably spend two and a half to three hours of my shift chasing up patient notes.

2.4.3   Communication Load

By illustrating the communication networks of clinicians in patient care, the complexity of the work of emergency clinicians becomes visible—we see how they diagnose and manage a patient during his or her stay in the emergency department. Time passed, shifts changed, handovers took place, information was incorrect or was lost, case notes were taken away and returned and then were lost again and equipment failed. Continuity of care was challenged as different clinicians attend to patients, and their consultations were interrupted and subjected to the vagaries of space, staffing resources and equipment failure. All of these events had potentially adverse consequences and emphasised the fragility of the *complex knowledge networks* of care surrounding the patients.

2.4.4   Communication Burden

Because clinicians change frequently and make limited use of written documentation, patients may be questioned repeatedly by different clinicians. For example, here is the same patient being questioned by three emergency department staff:

Triage nurse

Nurse 1: My name's Lorraine. Now tell me what's actually happened.
Patient: On Friday I was picking up the kids from my sister's place at about 4 or 5 and I tripped on, it was one step, and I tripped on the outdoor rubber mat 'cause I had heels on.

Doctor

Doctor 1: My name is Tatiana, one of the doctors here. How can I help you?
Patient: I've hurt my ribs ... that's all.
Doctor 1: Ah-hm. Do you remember how and when was that?
Patient: It was on Friday.

Nurse 4

Nurse 4: Did you have a fall or something or what happened?
Patient: On Friday I fell down—tripped on a mat, outdoor mat.==
Nurse 4: == OK.

We understand that the benefits of recursive questioning are that clinicians can check information straight from the source and can jog the patient's memory if required. Further, we recognise that asynchronous bedside attendances and recursive questioning are systemic and historical in origin and a feature of the way the emergency department is set up physically. They are a part of the way care takes place across space and time, rather than being indicative of ineffective practice by individual clinicians.

The benefits of this historical approach may outweigh the communication burden this created for the patient, who had to respond several times to the same or similar questions in one consultation. However, patient reports indicate that this recursive questioning can be seen as redundant and may even undermine patient confidence in clinicians. The exhausted and anxious patient can be left wondering why there appears to be no shared knowledge between clinicians. Most patients are not aware—and are not made aware by staff—that the emergency department is a training ground. Patients therefore do not appreciate the need for different clinicians to ask the same questions. Clearer explanations to patients, plus better quality written notes so that the senior doctor does not need to start the examination completely from scratch, would reduce this burden on the patient.

2.4.5   Communication Challenges of Multidisciplinary Care

Emergency departments are multidisciplinary healthcare sites, with major disciplinary divisions between nurses and doctors. Our observations, interviews and audio recordings suggest that while the disciplines work side by side, in all but one emergency department, there was very little interdisciplinary collaboration where greater role-blurring or sharing may occur (Opie 2000). In most cases, we saw clinicians attending the bedside individually and asynchronously, undertaking discipline-specific tasks and care.

While there may be good reasons for this differentiated practice (such as space limitations in cubicles or in circumstances where 'cross talk' between clinicians could confuse patients), separate care did mean that certain bits of information about the patient were segmented, which in some circumstances posed risks to patient safety. This occurred in Denton's case. Throughout his emergency department care, one of the questions about him that the clinicians were trying to solve is whether he was a CO_2 retainer (i. e. whether he retains carbon dioxide and should therefore not be given pure oxygen). When he was first admitted to the emergency department, Denton's old notes were not with him. They were brought into the emergency department relatively early in his stay, but at a number of points the notes went missing, presumably taken away by a clinician. Equipment was also a problem on the day, with a faulty ECG machine going offline. Clinicians expressed confusion about Denton's status as a CO_2 retainer on six separate occasions between 12:55 pm and 16:15 pm:

(1) 12:55 pm Nurse 2: We don't know if he's a CO_2 retainer?

(2) 14.00 pm Nurse in charge: Don't know too much about him.
(3) 14.25 pm Nurse 5: I don't know much about him but collapse, wasn't it?
(4) 14.30 pm Nurse 5: Is he—he's not a retainer, is he?
(5) 16:08 pm Doctor 1(Junior Medical Officer): Yes, I think he's a CO_2 retainer ...
(6) 16:15 pm Doctor 2 (senior staff specialist): No, because he's not a CO_2 retainer.
   So remember the gases. Got his old notes there? Remember I said if you look at
   the bicarb, that tells you what he's a CO_2 retainer. He's got normal bicarb so ...

Example 1 is nurse 2, talking to the ambulance officer. She admits that staff members do not know if Denton has this condition, which would suggest the need to find out but it does not get followed-up on. Nor does the nurse in charge (example 2) follows up. In examples 1, 2 and 3, the three different clinicians all use the same expression (*don't know*) to register their lack of knowledge about the patient's history and condition. This is further queried by nurse 5, the temporary relief nurse covering the lunch shift, in example (4), when she now presumes that *he is not a retainer*. The first doctor to see Denton (3 hrs into his emergency department stay), a Junior Medical Officer (JMO), picks up on this lack of knowledge but makes no definitive comment (*I think he is a CO_2 retainer*) as he did not know what the bicarb reading meant and only understood that Denton was not a retainer after this was explained to him by the senior Doctor. So it was only when the senior staff specialist (D2) arrived at 4:15 pm that a definite opinion was given when he directed the JMO to the patient's notes and explained what the bicarb reading meant.

This example demonstrates not only the risks to patients of discontinuous care by so many different clinicians but also the failure of the clinicians to collaborate: no one resolves the issue and no one provides this key information to subsequent clinicians.

In contrast, when we did see clinicians attending the bedside together, whether this was across disciplines or within disciplines (say between junior and senior doctors) it appeared to provide a greater and more efficient spread of the patient's story.

The high pace of work and increasing demands on their time mean that emergency department staff have few opportunities for cross-disciplinary handover, briefings or professional development. Many emergency departments hold no joint handovers or meetings, and nurses often complain about not being able to find doctors' notes. Separate care means segmentation of patient information. This translates to a potential risk to patient safety. The example with the patient Denton, discussed above, where nurses and doctors do not raise with each other the need to clarify Denton's CO_2 retainer status, is one example of a potentially serious failure of staff to take an interdisciplinary approach to the patient.

The sequential nature of clinical attendance also meant that patients responded consecutively to a number of unknown clinicians—this reinforced the rapid, changing and often fragmented or disrupted nature of the consultation. This information could and did easily become fragmented and nonlinear.

2.4.6   The Patient as Outsider: The Importance of Explanations

The patient remains an outsider to the institutionalised language and patterns of behaviour practised by emergency department staff. This can result in anxiety, informational incomprehension and/ or interpersonal alienation. While patients are often given key information and explanations about the processes of the emergency department and their situation, this is not always fully comprehended. Because of illnesses, anxiety and the way in which information is presented (in complex technical and institutional language), their understanding is often limited and fragmented. Hospital staff members recognise that while it is a stated priority to provide clear information to patients, it is not easy to do so because of time and clinical pressures (and of course the medical and/or mental condition of the patient). The following exchange between a young female patient and a doctor illustrates the patient's lack of familiarity with hospital practices—language and/or procedures:

Doctor: Might even ( ) Um, I think given that you're having a scan, a CAT scan, um,
  at some stage today.
Patient: Alright.
Doctor: But I'll keep you informed.
Patient: ( )
Doctor: Alright?
Patient: Did you get all that? [to the researcher]
(recorded in a consultation room)

This patient later made the comment 'I heard what she said but I don't know what she said' after the nurse told her what was about to happen.

The term computerised axial tomography (CAT) *scan* as well as the routine procedure of having one may have been new to the patient. Soon after, the patient commented 'Everyone tells you a different thing' after being told she was being admitted to the hospital for follow-up procedures; her comment demonstrates confusion regarding the interactions she has been involved in.

One emergency department director expressed the view that clinicians often make the mistake of thinking that patients understand all the explanations they are given and underestimate the effect that the emergency department context can have on an individual patient's ability to comprehend what is happening to them—on younger patients, because the emergency department is generally unfamiliar, and on older patients, because they may have hearing or cognitive difficulties, or be seriously ill.

> I think that one of the key things with communication in the Emergency Department is a realisation of how little patients can actually retain, even though we seem to think that they really have got it. And they think—and in fairness, they think they really have got it. But they haven't and I think we make that mistake over and over and over again ... For many people it's overwhelming partly because it's complex but because people are pretty generally healthy. There's not—you know, young people under the age of 65 are not overly familiar with medical care, hospital care and the older people that we see who are very familiar, they have other issues. They have cognitive issues, they have hearing issues. And they have more severe medical illnesses (director of an emergency department).

The examples below with Wilson (sore toe) and Dulcie (difficulty breathing: discussed above), occur at slightly different points in their admission stages. The more
experienced nurse in Wilson's case has a good grasp of what patients want to know,
whereas the new graduate nurse who interacts with Dulcie provides very little information about what will come next in her care. We contrast the two examples to
illustrate how a senior nurse has developed both awareness of what patients want
to know and skills in how to let them know what is happening. She combined this
awareness and skill with a systematic approach to explaining to patients what the
emergency department process was about. In the less effective example, with Dulcie, the new graduate nurse focused intently on his own protocols, provided very
little future-signposted information and forgot to follow-up on Dulcie's request for
a bed warmer.

More effective (Wilson)	Less effective (Dulcie)
Nurse: [Siren in background while nurse 2 is talking]. Yes. I've got a form here for you. It's to enable you to understand what's going on with you while you're here. OK? So you fill it out when you know who your nurse is and what your doctor's name is, what tests you've had or what tests you're waiting for or what medication you're waiting for, things like that so you know ... so you're not just sitting there going 'What's going on'? [Family member laughing at the siren] Alright? Whether you can eat and drink, you know, those sorts of things. So they're the sorts of things that you ask, and you can fill that out if you want. [Fire alarm is tested—this happens as Nurse 2 is talking] *Patient: OK.* *Nurse: Or the nurse will fill it out.* *Patient: Alright.* *Nurse: So ask her what her name is* *Patient: OK.* *Nurse: And just so you know what's going on so you're not sitting here ==* *Patient: == Yup ==* *Nurse: == Going 'I wonder what's happening?'* *Patient: [Chuckles]. Alright, then.* *Nurse: So what is happening is that you're waiting for your nurse to come over and introduce herself but she's a little bit tied up so she'll be with you as soon as == she can.*	*Nurse: Hi I'm Sandy, I'm a nurse.* *Patient: How are you?* *Nurse: Good thanks.* *Nurse: OK. So your full name please?* *Patient: Dulcie [surname].* *Nurse: Lovely. And your date of birth please?* *Patient: [DOB]. ==* *Nurse: == Terrific. Alright. Just lie down on the bed for me please, Dulcie. [Patient coughs]* *.............[Nurse leaves to get armband]* *Nurse: OK. So I'll just ask you again, Dulcie, for your full name please.* *Patient: Dulcie [surname].* *Nurse: And your date of birth please?* *Patient: [DOB]* *Nurse: Thank you.* *Patient: I'll get the six out yet. Twice I've had a shot at that.* *Nurse: Alright.* *....................* *Nurse: You in any pain at all Dulcie?* *Patient: No. Me feet are frozen, I don't know why.* *Nurse: OK.* *Patient: Oh, gawd.* *Nurse: I'll keep that in mind. [chuckles]* *Patient: Need a bed warmer.* *Nurse: Be back soon. [Nurse 2 leaves at 12.03 pm, returns at 12.35 pm]*

More effective (Wilson)	Less effective (Dulcie)
In this example, the nurse, one of the admitting nurses, explained to Wilson (sore toe), how to complete a 'patient progress' form. After explaining this to Wilson, which took a considerable time, she then proceeded to tell him where he was up to in his care and importantly, what would happen next. A little while later Nurse 2, who also looked after Wilson, was impressed to see the sheets were being of some, but limited use: *Nurse 2: You know Wilson, you're one of the very few that have actually filled one of those out, I'm very impressed*	*In this example, the nurse has a very different approach to his experienced counterpart in the more effective example. He is a new graduate nurse and comes into the room with a pad and writes notes as he speaks to Dulcie (difficulty breathing). The nurse is very focused on protocols (institutional knowledge—getting the patient's name and date of birth correct etc.). His introduction is very different to the norm of what we have recorded. Nurse 2 gives his professional role without any institutional affiliation, 'I'm Sandy. I'm a nurse'. Shortly after that he has to get an armband—and when he returns two minutes later, he focuses again on the protocols of rechecking Dulcie's name and date of birth and re-asks her for these details. A little later on, he does not explain why he wants Dulcie to lie down, and when Dulcie says her feet are cold, he says 'I'll keep that in mind'. He leaves without any explanation of what processes will come next, does not bring the bed warmer and returns half an hour later. He gives Dulcie no explanation about what will happen next. He leaves her confused about whether or not he is coming back. Dulcie said after he left 'Ah, well I think he's coming back isn't ==* *he'? The nurse's focus was on institutional protocols and his communication was formulaic*

2.4.7   Different Understandings of Time

Time plays a central role in the way the emergency department works, both as a resource and as a phenomenon experienced by patients and healthcare practitioners. Elapsed time (waiting) can have a significant impact on the overall patient experience. Recordings of consultations and our observations revealed that references to time, by doctors in particular, ranged from the abstract to the numerically specific, for example, 'I won't be long' to 'I'll be back in 10 minutes' (a specific time frame was often found to be unrealistic). Often patients did not have a clear understanding of how long a procedure would take, or how long an absence would be. Sometimes the patient quickly recognised the elasticity of time. For example, one patient said, 'When they say time [they will be away], I think it's a figure of speech for them', and later articulated a similar idea through the statement 'Meanwhile the doctor's gone to lunch' when the doctor was called away from the consultation room.

Additionally, consultations between patients and doctors are often interrupted. Sometimes the interruption lasts only for a few seconds as the doctor can be called away via his or her beeper. The following exchange between an elderly male patient and a male doctor occurred only a minute or two after the consultation had started:

Doctor: I've been caught up in something else
Patient: Yes?
Doctor: I'll be with you though ==
Patient: That's all right
Doctor: == in about 5–10 min
Patient: Yeah, right-o

The doctor returned half an hour later. During the subsequent consultation, the same patient was interrupted a number of times when the doctor was called out to attend to another patient—a regular occurrence for senior doctors.

Notably, none of the participants (clinicians or patients) in the consultations that we recorded had any real control over their own time and the time taken for medical analyses. This produced very different behaviour on the part of clinicians and patients. Our observations showed that many clinicians and patients in the emergency department operated with competing time frames. While doctors moved quickly, frequently interrupting consultations to attend to other emergencies as required by the exigent nature of the emergency department, patients had little choice but to *wait*, and nurses attempted to mediate between the fast pace of medical attention and the stasis imposed on patients. Patients were obliged to wait in the waiting room, to wait on test results, information, diagnosis, disposition and bed placement, with little explanation as to why this was happening or when things would occur.

Added to our observations, recorded comments by patients showed how the potential discord resulting from different perceptions of time could poorly affect a patient's overall experience in the emergency department. Attentive to the organisational implications of these competing goals, the nurse's priority is continuity of flow, even if it is rarely achieved:

> [My role] 'primarily being patient flow ... because obviously flow is very important ... So it's very important to try and, you know identify where there's potential for bottlenecks and fast tracking patients ...' (nursing unit manager)

One clinician—an intern (interview: hospital A)—summed this up very well when he said:

> It's really bad because ... in a lot of ways, because there's so many delays and while I'm very, very busy... My interactions with one individual patient might be hours apart. And so for that one patient, even though I feel like everything's happening, when you sort of think about it you realise that they've been sitting in that bed with nothing happening for hours and hours. So I think there's ... I mean there's lots of reasons for the delays and there's a delay sort of from presenting to actually coming into the department, and there's delays from coming in and actually being seen by a doctor and then they get seen by a doctor who sort of comes and asks them lots of questions, pokes and prods them and then disappears for hours and hours while blood tests come back and X-rays happen and all that sort of thing. So I often think... yeah I don't... I think I would have to be seriously ill to go to an ED (laughter) just because I think it would be such a frustrating experience and particularly late at night because it never closes down... The lights are always on, there's always noise and there's always people and I think if I felt like that person probably feels, the last thing I would want would be a big noisy room with people running around and no one coming when I press my button and... so that sort of thing. So I think it's a very frustrating and prolonged experience for them.

2.5   Conclusion

In Fig. 2.5 below, we summarise our contextual characterisation of emergency departments and the impact of these features on the nature of communication in emergency departments. In the next chapter, we present a brief summary of what goes on

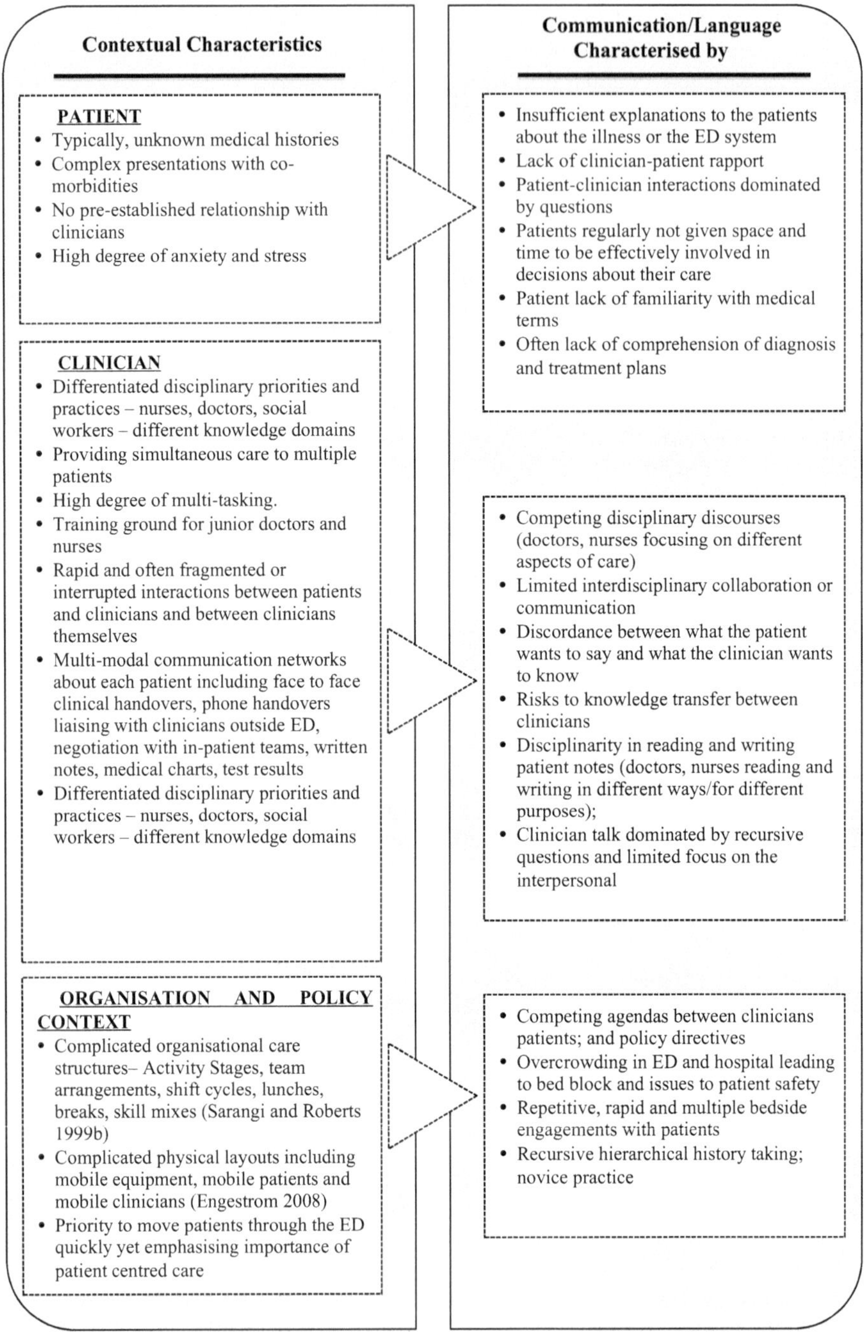

Contextual Characteristics

PATIENT
- Typically, unknown medical histories
- Complex presentations with co-morbidities
- No pre-established relationship with clinicians
- High degree of anxiety and stress

CLINICIAN
- Differentiated disciplinary priorities and practices – nurses, doctors, social workers – different knowledge domains
- Providing simultaneous care to multiple patients
- High degree of multi-tasking.
- Training ground for junior doctors and nurses
- Rapid and often fragmented or interrupted interactions between patients and clinicians and between clinicians themselves
- Multi-modal communication networks about each patient including face to face clinical handovers, phone handovers liaising with clinicians outside ED, negotiation with in-patient teams, written notes, medical charts, test results
- Differentiated disciplinary priorities and practices – nurses, doctors, social workers – different knowledge domains

ORGANISATION   AND   POLICY CONTEXT
- Complicated organisational care structures– Activity Stages, team arrangements, shift cycles, lunches, breaks, skill mixes (Sarangi and Roberts 1999b)
- Complicated physical layouts including mobile equipment, mobile patients and mobile clinicians (Engestrom 2008)
- Priority to move patients through the ED quickly yet emphasising importance of patient centred care

Communication/Language Characterised by

- Insufficient explanations to the patients about the illness or the ED system
- Lack of clinician-patient rapport
- Patient-clinician interactions dominated by questions
- Patients regularly not given space and time to be effectively involved in decisions about their care
- Patient lack of familiarity with medical terms
- Often lack of comprehension of diagnosis and treatment plans

- Competing disciplinary discourses (doctors, nurses focusing on different aspects of care)
- Limited interdisciplinary collaboration or communication
- Discordance between what the patient wants to say and what the clinician wants to know
- Risks to knowledge transfer between clinicians
- Disciplinarity in reading and writing patient notes (doctors, nurses reading and writing in different ways/for different purposes);
- Clinician talk dominated by recursive questions and limited focus on the interpersonal

- Competing agendas between clinicians patients; and policy directives
- Overcrowding in ED and hospital leading to bed block and issues to patient safety
- Repetitive, rapid and multiple bedside engagements with patients
- Recursive hierarchical history taking; novice practice

Fig. 2.5 The contextual and communicative complexity of the emergency department

behaviourally and linguistically in each of the stages of the patient journey through the emergency department, and the particular challenges and risks involved in each stage.

References

Australian Institute of Health and Welfare (2013). *Australian hospital statistics 2012–13: Emergency department care*. Canberra: AIHW.

Bernstein, S. L., Aronsky, D., Duseja, R., et al. (2009). The effect of emergency department crowding on clinically oriented outcomes. *Academic Emergency Medicine, 16*, 1–10.

Coiera, E. W., Jayasuriya, R. A., Hardy, J., Bannan, A., & Thorpe, M. E. C. (2002). Communication loads on clinical staff in the emergency department. *Medical Journal of Australia, 176*, 415–418.

Committee on the Future of Emergency Care in the United States Health System. (2006). *Hospital-based emergency care: At the breaking point*. Washington DC: National Academies Press.

Crawford, K., Morphet, J., Jones, T., Innes, K., Griffiths, D., & Williams, A. (2013). Initiatives to reduce overcrowding and access block in Australian emergency departments: A literature review. *Collegian*. doi:10.1016/j.colegn.2013.09.005.

Durand, A., Palazzolo, S., Tanti-Hardouin, N., Gerbeaux, P., Sambuc, R., & Gentile, S. (2012). Nonurgent patients in emergency departments: Rational or irresponsible consumers? Perceptions of professionals and patients. *BMC Research Notes, 5*, 525.

Eggins, S., & Slade, D. (2012). Clinical handover as an interactive event: Informational and interactional communication strategies in effective shift-change handovers. *Communication & Medicine, 9*(3), 215–227.

Eggins, S., & Slade, D. (forthcoming). *Effective Communication in Clinical Handover—Research and Practice* De Gruyter Mouton, Berlin; (PASA, Patient Safety 16).

Fairbanks, R. J., Bisantz, A. M., & Sunm, M. (2007). Emergency department communication links and patterns. *Annals of Emergency Medicine, 50*, 396–406. doi:10.1016/j.annemergmed.2007.03.005.

Garling, P. (2008). *Final report of the Special Commission of Inquiry: Acute Care Services in NSW Public Hospitals* (Vols. 1–2). Sydney: Special Commission of Inquiry.

Kee, R. S., Knott, J. C., Dreyfus, S., Lederman, R., Milton, S., & Joe, K. (2012). One hundred tasks an hour: An observational study of emergency department consultant activities. *Emergency Medicine Australasia, 24*(3), 294–302. doi:10.1111/j.1742-6723.2012.01540.x.

Lowthian, J., Curtis, A., Jolley, D., Stoelwinder, J., McNeil, J., & Cameron, P. (2012). Demand at the emergency department front door: 10-year trends in presentations. *Medical Journal of Australia, 196*(2), 128–132.

Manidis, M. (2013). 'Practising knowing in emergency departments: Tracing the disciplinary and institutional complexities of working, learning and knowing in emergency departments'. PhD thesis, University of Technology Sydney.

Manidis, M., Slade, D., McGregor, J., Chandler, E., Dunston, R., Scheeres, H., Stein-Parbury, J., Iedema, R., & Stanton, N. (2009). *Emergency communication: report for Prince of Wales Hospital*. Sydney: University of Technology Sydney.

Navin, M., & Sacco, W. (2010). Science and evidence-based considerations for fulfilling the SALT triage framework. *Disaster Medicine and Public Health Preparedness, 4*(1), 10–12.

Opie, L. (2000). *Drugs and the Heart* (5th ed.). London: WB Saunders.

Perez-Carceles, M., Gironda, J., Osuna, E., Falcon, M., & Luna, A. (2010). Is the right to information fulfilled in an emergency department? Patients' perceptions of the care provided. *Journal of Evaluation in Clinical Practice, 16,* 456–463.

Redfern, E., Brown, R., & Vincent, C. A. (2009). Identifying vulnerabilities in communication in the emergency department. *Emergency Medicine Journal, 26*(9), 653–657.

Schatzki, T. (2011). Where the Action Is (On Large Social Phenomena Such as Sociotechnical Regimes). Sustainable Practices Research Group Working Paper 1. http://www.sprg.ac.uk/uploads/schatzki-wp1.pdf. Accessed 17 Oct 2014

Schull, M. J., Slaughter, P. M., & Redelmeier, D. A. (2002). Urban emergency department overcrowding: Defining the problem and eliminating misconceptions. *Canadian Journal of Emergency Medicine, 4*(2), 76–83.

Short, A. E., Short, K. T., Holdgate, A., Ahern, N., & Morris, J. (2011). Noise levels in an Australian emergency department. *Australasian Emergency Nursing Journal, 14,* 26–31. doi:10.1016/j.aenj.2010.10.005.

Slade, D., Manidis, M., McGregor, J., Scheeres, H., Stein-Parbury, J., Dunston, R., Stanton, N., Chandler, E., Matthiessen, C., & Herke, M. (2011). *Communicating in hospital emergency departments. Final report* (Vol 1). Sydney: University of Technology Sydney.

Spencer, R., Coiera, E., & Logan, P. (2004). Variation in communication loads on clinical staff in the emergency department. *Annals of Emergency Medicine, 44*(3), 268–273. doi:org/10.1016/j.annemergmed.2004.04.006.

Woloshynowych, M., Davis, R., Brown, R., & Vincent, C. (2007). Communication patterns in a UK emergency department. *Annals of Emergency Medicine, 50*(4), 407–413. doi:10.1016/j.annemergmed.2007.08.001.

Chapter 3
The Patient's Journey in the Emergency Department from Triage to Disposition

3.1 Introduction

Two main priorities guide emergency department care. The first is to determine a patient's diagnosis. The second is to determine whether that patient can be safely treated within the emergency department and discharged home, or whether they need to be admitted for further treatment and supervision in another hospital ward or health-care facility. From the moment patients arrive at the emergency department to the point of their disposition, their care becomes organised systematically into a series of activities (what we refer to as 'activity stages'—derived from Engestrom's 2008 work on systems), each with their own short-term clinical goals, sequentially driven to achieve these outcomes.

In this chapter, we present a brief summary of what goes on behaviourally and linguistically during each activity stage. Our descriptions are interspersed with vignettes from researcher observation notes and excerpts from interviews with staff, illustrating the multidisciplinary dynamics and challenges associated with each stage.

By dividing the sequence of activities, patients go through a limited number of activity stages; we can effectively describe the issues and challenges at each stage through the patient's journey. Emergency department consultations in the adult section of the department with patients who are categorised at triage levels 3–5 (that is, they do not require immediate medical attention) can be divided into four broad activity stages, based on four distinct divisions of labour and responsibility. Within each activity stage, there is a strong emphasis on discipline-specific practice and communication, and team activity generally consists of parallel disciplinary activity. In the third stage, we see more evidence of teams that connect horizontally, across disciplinary boundaries. The four activity stages are:

- Triage
- Nursing admission

© Springer-Verlag Berlin Heidelberg 2015
D. Slade et al., *Communicating in Hospital Emergency Departments,*
DOI 10.1007/978-3-662-46021-4_3

- Initial medical consultation—initial contact, exploration of condition, history-taking, diagnostic tests and procedures
- Final medical consultation—diagnosis, treatment and disposition.

Our account of emergency department activity stages begins with *triage*. This marks the first encounter patients have with emergency department staff and the point at which an assessment is made concerning the urgency of their presenting condition. We then describe the *nursing admission* process, when patients are moved beyond the waiting room, inside the emergency department and monitored by nurses as they wait to be seen by a doctor. When the doctor appears, this generally marks the beginning of the patient's medical consultation. A resident (junior) doctor, who usually does the initial assessment during the *initial medical consultation*, takes the patient's history, performs a physical exam and organises tests to help determine the patient's diagnosis. After the patient's test results come through, a *final medical consultation* takes place, at which point a more senior doctor typically appears at the patient's bedside. During this activity stage the patient's diagnosis is confirmed, a treatment plan is negotiated, and a decision is made in relation to the patient's disposition.

As we describe each of the typical stages of the emergency department patient's journey below, we begin with an account of its function, and follow this with a description of the typical communication patterns of the stage. (In Chaps. 5 and 6, we describe in greater detail the characteristic communicative features of effective and less-effective interactions). We show how, at different points, the composition of the clinical team which appears beside the patient changes, and different disciplines (nursing or medical) take primary responsibility, or work side by side with each other, at times with competing immediate care priorities. Each stage is associated with predictable and highly constrained communication choices and produces particular patterns in clinician–patient communication. Together, the stages shape the patient's emergency department experience.

3.2   Triage

Triage is the first stage of patient care in the emergency department after the patient arrives through the waiting room or the ambulance bay. During this stage, a nurse assesses the urgency of a patient's presenting condition. In the emergency departments we studied, triage assessments usually occurred in a small consulting room allocated specifically for that purpose or at the triage window, using a uniform set of criteria to categorise patients into one of five categories according to urgency and acuity. Many triage interviews were audible from the waiting room or the triage window.

Each hospital emergency department had slightly different approaches to triage. In some, triage nurses worked in pairs or were assisted by others who liaised with other clinicians. Patients with obvious injuries, such as broken bones, were sent for an X-ray before a doctor saw them. In other hospitals, if a patient was identified at

Table 3.1 Triage systems in the five emergency departments studied

Hospital A	Hospital B	Hospital C	Hospital D	Hospital E
Two nurses work in tandem in two different rooms	One nurse works with an assistant in nursing (AIN) or junior 'runner'	Nurses work in pairs in one space; queues can be lengthy at times	Two or three nurses work in one space; very busy	Nurses work in pairs, one in ambulance bay, the other at window; very small room

triage as needing a bed, the triage nurse(s) negotiated with the nursing team leader who allocated beds in the emergency department when they became available. The different approaches we observed are summarised in Table 3.1.

3.2.1 Waiting Room

Our observations of goings-on in the waiting room were similar across the five emergency departments we visited. At peak times (between 11 am and 11 pm), many of the seats were taken. At other times (for example, 8 am–9 am), the waiting rooms were virtually empty. In most cases, signs directed patients to the triage nurse for assessment. More urgent cases were taken straight into the emergency department. The rest were asked to register their details (name, date of birth, marital status, etc.) with the clerical staff outside in the waiting room, and then to take a seat until a doctor could see them.

The amount of written information available to inform patients about the emergency department process, particularly the triage system and how long it could take before they were admitted for emergency department care, was variable across the five emergency departments. However, on the whole very little information was provided. In all emergency departments, patients tended to return to the triage nurse to get updates on waiting times. Some patients were extremely nervous about entering the 'visual space' of the triage nurse; triage nurses themselves were frequently so busy that they chose not to (or did not) 'see' the patients or carers who reapproached them.

Observation Field Notes in a Waiting Room, 2 pm

Over 30 people are in the waiting room. One person with a suspected deep vein thrombosis (DVT) goes up to the window at 14.05. She says she has been waiting for 4 hrs. She wants to go home, her husband says, 'No, we are not going home'. An emergency department (ED) doctor brings out a letter and gives it to a patient. People are reading absentmindedly, turning pages. Hospital staff walks through. One man returns to the waiting room from an outside call at 14.10. Someone drops a radio, checks it is still working. A wheelchair is wheeled through at 14.14. A sleeping elderly woman wakes up when a trolley is banged next door. A man in a wheelchair is wheeled through. Another man is trying to sleep on a wheelchair. At 14.18 a new person is called in to the ED. A man with his arm in a sling, accompanied by two people, walks through. A woman on crutches walks through. At 14.27 someone places a blanket on a girl in a wheelchair. People pick up books, babies are squealing; the ED doctor calls in a new person to see at 14.37. One woman is on a mobile phone; some are flipping through magazines; some are just looking; one young man is balancing on crutches; a patient exits from fast track. The carer with the woman who has suspected DVT goes up to the window at 15.08 to say 'We are not going to wait'.

Some patients and carers exhibited high levels of anxiety and frustration in the waiting room, particularly after they had been left unattended in the waiting room for a considerable amount of time. Occasionally, a nurse ventured out to let the patients know how long they would be waiting, or to administer an analgesic. These interventions when they occurred were very warmly received. Triage nurses, however, were frequently limited in the amount of information they gave patients about waiting times, and what would happen in the next stage of their journey. The exchange below exemplifies this. It took place at 11.24 am on a particularly busy day.

The triage nurse had just ventured out of the consultation room to conduct observations of patients in the waiting room. One patient, Jack (MS, feeling unwell, weak), had been waiting for admission to the emergency department since 9 am. When the triage nurse approached Jack, she immediately advised Jack that because more sick people had presented to the emergency department since he had arrived, he would have to wait longer before seeing a doctor:

> *Nurse 1: Yes, so we have just had a couple of people who have come in.*
> *Patient: Okay.*
> *Nurse 1: So a little bit more urgent at this point.*
> *Patient: No worries.*
> *Nurse 1: But it's churning along, it's always this time.*
> *Patient: Yeah, no worries. We …*
> *Nurse 1: How are you feeling right now?*
> *Patient: Oh, still lousy but …*
> *Nurse 1: Yeah. Worse?*
> *Patient: Oh, about the same. [Pause in talking, distant background noises, approx one minute while N1 does obs]*
> *Patient: Okay? Can I just …?*
> *Nurse 1: That's all.*
> *Patient: Oh, good. Thank = = you for that.*
> *Nurse 1: = = Fine, looks good. And so, yeah, we'll just let you know how it's going = = I guess.*
> *Patient: = = Yeah. You see, no—no time frame? You don't …?*
> *Nurse 1: No, sorry.*
> *Patient: That's alright. Thank you.*

This interaction illustrates how difficult it is for triage nurses to give time frames for waiting patients. It also shows, after the explanation, Jack's willingness to accept this reality: 'That's alright. Thank you'.

3.2.2   Ambulance Bays

Patients who arrived at the emergency department by ambulance were triaged while they were still on the ambulance trolley. The ambulance officer would give medical details of the presentation to the triage nurse, who would then categorise the patient for treatment, following the same uniform set of criteria used for walk-in patients. Triage nurses occasionally initiated treatment (in the form of pain relief, for example) to patients while they were waiting in the ambulance bay. Ambulance bays could get extremely hectic, as the following observation notes show:

Observation Field Notes from the Ambulance Bay, 1.30 pm

There is a very elderly, frail patient on a trolley. A female ambulance officer is handing over to the triage nurse. The patient has recently increased medication to help with cramping and is not able to communicate normally. His elderly wife (hunched with a walking stick) is with him. Two male ambulance officers are standing by. The triage nurse knows the patient and the ambulance officers. We can hear a baby crying from one of the cubicles. The patient is taken to bed 6. The baby is still crying. A man is wheeled into Triage, speaking to the triage nurse who is taking 'obs'. An elderly female patient is wheeled from bed 19 to? There is laughter from the 'station'. Another male at Triage is being given 'obs' and he then goes back to waiting room. A woman with a baby arrives at the triage window who then comes through into Triage; we overhear the word 'diarrhoea'. The male patient on a wheelchair leaves Triage to return to the waiting room. A male patient, 54 years, is brought in by male and female ambulance officers. They check his pulse and blood pressure. They hand over to the triage nurse—suspected anaphylactic reaction to medication (penicillin). The patient has previously had pleurisy and pneumonia. The patient has had shaking, shortness of breath and redness to body. The triage nurse says, 'We will get you seen to straight away'. The patient is taken to bed 4.

Another ambulance arrives and then another. An elderly female patient had a fall at the hostel this morning and then came over all hot and clammy. She felt fine to go out for lunch at the RSL with her husband where she took a turn for the worse. She appear to be very disorientated. The triage nurse asks her what month it is which she knows but not what year it is. The ambulance officers are told to take her to bed 16 but someone is already there. She is wheeled to the corridor. She smells as if she has defecated.

An elderly male patient, Sam, aged 99, arrives. He lives at home alone; had a fall this morning and cut his head. The triage nurse feels his arm, 'you are cold darling'. Sam does not take any medication except two lite beers a day. The triage nurse, 'You are amazing, you have got ages to go yet'. Sam used to be a butcher.

Now there are seven ambulance officers standing around laughing and joking. There seems to be a real camaraderie with the ED staff.

Another ambulance arrives with a 61-year-old man who dropped his hands into 90° hot wax.

Another ambulance arrives with an elderly male in a wheelchair. All the ambulance officers know him; he seems to be a regular to the ED. A drinker. Apparently he had rung an ambulance several times the previous night; it seems they only pick him up if they are not too busy.

3.2.3   Communication in the Triage Stage

In the triage stage, the major communicative responsibilities fall to the triage nurse who will interview patients about their symptoms and medical history, in order to assess the patients accurately and subsequently assign them an appropriate triage category. The importance of the triage nurse in the emergency department communication network is highlighted by the following comment from a member of the clerical team:

> Good communication is when the triage nurse and us are on the same wavelength. If the triage nurse is happy then we're happy, then the doctor's happy. Everything's running smoothly. (Communication supervisor)

Clinicians we interviewed frequently remarked that if there were misunderstandings or errors of communication between the patient and the triage nurse, this would have a ripple effect throughout the patient's journey.

The triage stage is characteristically brief and the role of the triage nurse is clearly prescribed. The triage nurse must balance a number of competing priorities during his or her assessment process, including the medical priority of patient care, the organisational priority of allocating the correct category and the most appropriate assessment/treatment area, and the professional priority of performing discipline-specific practice, which includes being accountable for these decisions. In Australia, triage nurses are senior nurses who are specially trained to assess patients. As an advanced practice nurse described, one of the main communication challenges for triage nurses is to sift out the clinically relevant information from patient descriptions of their symptoms and what led them to seek care in the emergency department, 'because often what the patient says to triage and what they have actually got wrong with them are two totally different things' (advanced practice nurse).

The interview between the nurse and the patient during the triage assessment is framed by a uniform set of criteria designed to make the process both thorough and efficient. During the brief encounter, patients are asked to provide limited information in response to a very specific series of questions and are not encouraged to ask questions of their own. Patients are invited to tell their story succinctly and coherently. If they do not do this, the triage nurse intervenes to achieve the goals of the triage consultation. An excerpt from one triage consultation with Natasha (post-op infection due to a breast augmentation), demonstrates how the nurse elicits crucial information:

Patient: And then today I started to really feel unwell and I feel like it's a heart attack actually. Just really sharp pains in my chest and my left breast is swollen () fever, gone down my arm, you know ...
Nurse: Okay, so it's particularly the left one.
Patient: It's the = = right one ...
Nurse: And = = () swollen, or ...
Patient: Yep, yep, and that's where all the pain is.
Nurse: Okay. And how long has that been like that for?
Patient: The pain has been since I had the op, but it's ...
Nurse: Okay, but the swelling and the ...

The overall structure of the interactions we found in most triage consultations was very similar, despite differences in the levels of medical complexity of patient presentations. The agenda was clearly set by the triage nurse, and interactions were characteristically short. For example, in Jean's case (Jean presented with minor leg trauma) the triage nurse asked nine questions: four were about the patient's presenting condition and five related to the organisational processes of the emergency department (we refer to this as the 'hospital system' from this point). The nurse also made three statements during the assessment process, all related to the hospital system. Jean asked no questions, and her contribution was limited to providing short, concise responses to the nurse's questions.

As stated above, the information patients receive is usually limited to what they can expect to happen until they are moved from the waiting room to a bed inside the emergency department. In other words, patients are generally not given an outline of what they can expect to happen during their overall emergency department journey. It is likely that patients initially find the triage/emergency department context bewildering, especially if they are in distress. The information triage nurses provide usually relates to approximate waiting times or refers, in general terms, to the staff members who will follow.

There is often little time in the triage stage for the nurse to establish a relationship with the patient. However, we noted that sometimes they managed to convey a positive friendly attitude by using a few simple strategies. They would, for example, establish rapport with the patient by introducing themselves informally and describing their role, use inclusive language and occasionally terms of endearment, and further give supportive or empathetic feedback to patients when they describe their pain or anxiety.

3.2.4   Communication in the Triage Stage: Summary

- Language is constrained by a uniform set of criteria and a clearly defined process.
- A limited number of prescribed questions are designed to achieve correct triage allocation.
- Patients are not encouraged to ask questions of their own.
- Patients rarely ask questions about what is going to happen to them beyond triage.
- The information patients receive is generally limited to what they can expect to happen until the end of this particular stage.

- The information triage nurses provide relates to approximate waiting times or to the staff members who will follow.
- There is limited opportunity to establish an interpersonal relationship.
- The important aspects of language and communication in triage are those that recognise the patient's unfamiliarity with the emergency department process and those that address their vulnerability in presenting to the emergency department. Actions which do this include clinicians greeting the patient and introducing themselves and their roles, allowing the patient to tell their story, normalising the patient's concerns, and explaining what will be happening next, including providing information about the entire process of the emergency department.

3.3 Nursing Admission

Following triage, patients will typically be asked to sit in the waiting room until they are admitted into the emergency department. Their admission, when it eventually takes place, will be handled by nurses who are allocated to patient beds in teams. The teams will usually consist of junior and senior nurses, with the former supervised by the latter as part of the process of situational learning. The nurses perform their own discipline-specific practice and are answerable to the hierarchy within their own discipline. Nurses responsible for the admission of patients have a clearly defined role. First, they perform the task of admitting patients in the emergency department, which involves getting patients changed into hospital gowns and recording their personal details. Second, they make sure that patients are medically stable by doing basic observations, recording information in patient notes and administering pain relief to patients when necessary. Handover to consecutive nursing staff is both written (patient notes) and spoken.

Throughout this stage, nurses need to balance the competing priorities of the organisation of the emergency department with the priority of patient care. Depending on the urgency of each patient's condition and the number of people the emergency department is dealing with, a number of different clinicians (nurses and junior and senior doctors) may surround the patient at the same time—or may simply pass by—during this stage. This can create a hectic, noisy atmosphere around the patient's bedside.

Observation Field Notes from Bed 3 in Acute, 3 pm

On this day 36 people have walked past the bed in a space of fifteen minutes, the fire alarms have been tested twice; on 24 occasions the noise was so high as to interfere with audible communication with the patient; there were 10 overhead announcements and/or code calls; and 180 patients have fronted up to the ED in the previous 24 hrs resulting in a very stressed set of interactions for all the clinicians concerned as well as for the patient. People going past the bed one after the other include one team leader, one carer, one person in a bed, one person in a wheelchair, two staff nurses, four doctors and two people with IV drips.

3.3.1 Communication in the Nursing Admission Stage

Communication in the nursing admission stage is challenged by three requirements: the need for nursing staff to manage and adapt their priorities according to changing demands, particularly in very busy times; the need for all clinicians to communicate effectively with the multidisciplinary team; and the need for nursing staff to attend to the disorientation patients experience in the emergency department. One senior nurse we interviewed summed up the priority for the nursing teams in the admission process:

> I like to package people to a degree. I like to get all their observations done and make sure they are settled, and their pain's under control, and all the pieces of paper that go along with it and my documentation. And then I can sort of think … I know everything that I could possibly know right now, until something [else happens]. I like to sort of go right; I know if I walk away for the next 10 min, it is all kind of sorted for you. (Clinical nurse specialist)

It is through nursing admission that patients enter the main clinical areas of the emergency department and become part of the hospital system, and many are highly anxious and feel a loss of personal control. Pain and distress contribute to the feeling of powerlessness, and this can be magnified by other factors such as gender, age and socioeconomic circumstances. Most clinicians we interviewed were aware of the emotional impact of hospitalisation on patients:

> No one wants to come to an emergency department so you're dealing with consumers who are distressed. So every single patient that we deal with has some form of stress and so that makes it a particularly different area to work in. (Nursing unit manager)

> I think it can be a very daunting experience. I think it can be quite scary sometimes … because they come in to what can be a foreign environment … so what concerns me is how they perceive how we treat other patients sometimes because, especially with our mental health patients who might need to be sedated and that sort of thing, I quite often think about what other patients may think what we're doing to these patients. (Staff nurse)

One way in which nurses can reduce patient anxiety is to keep them informed in terms of their treatment and also a propos the emergency department processes they will become involved in or will see around them. Patients may not always be well enough or confident enough to ask questions, or understand information provided.

The amount of time that nurses have with patients is a major limitation. A number of nurses we interviewed described how the interpersonal dimensions of providing care were frequently compromised by high patient loads. When the department is under pressure, nurses described having to prioritise their work differently, as they spread themselves across the needs of several patients simultaneously:

> Often there is a time factor where if the department's really busy and we're short staffed or you know the level of staffing isn't as it should be, then you start to run into problems where you need to just do the basics for one person and then move on to the next one because there just isn't time and if you sort of get three new patients all at once, you have to prioritise what your duties are. So I personally just go back to my basic nursing, make sure they've got observations, electrocardiogram (ECG) and you know make sure they're stable for the moment, then I'll move on and then come back, if there is time to do the more, you know, the higher skills, I guess. (Staff nurse)

The need to work at maximum pace meant that patients were given less time to ask and respond to questions. Many also got less information than they wanted about what would happen to them next, and when it would happen.

> Sometimes it's very organised and things go well. Sometimes I think we try to rush our patients through and not that we miss things, but sometimes I don't think we take a holistic approach. I think we just hone in [home in] on what's wrong with them, get them in, get them out and let someone else do the definitive care. I think sometimes we forget that we do actually complete definite care here sometimes. (Transitional nurse practitioner)

The language patterns we found during the admission stage of all patient journeys showed clear similarities and reflected the nurse's practice described above. We used a move analysis[1] (where we analyse the number and type of questions, statements and acknowledgements made by the nurses and patients) to examine the kinds of utterances made by nurses and patients in this stage. This analysis showed that the exchange of information between nurse and patient was often limited to a brief review of the presenting medical condition, and that the nurse would typically provide a series of statements to the patient concerning the emergency department processes associated with the admission stage. The patient's main contribution was through their answers to the nurse's questions. The overall emphasis in most patient admissions was on orienting patients about what they should expect to happen during admission, and preparing them for seeing a doctor in the next stage. Most often they announce the (pending) arrival of the doctor

3.3.2   Summary: Communication in Nursing Admission

- Patients rarely ask questions about what is going to happen to them.
- The information patients receive is generally limited to what they can expect to happen in this particular activity stage.
- There is limited opportunity to establish an interpersonal relationship (as the stage is very short), but often this is the first opportunity the nurses have to reassure the patients and calm their anxiety about being in the emergency department.
- The stage is dominated by nurses introducing the patient to the institutional life of the hospital. Nurses focus on protocols about the patient's allergies, personal identification, belongings, changing them into the hospital gowns, their comfort, etc.
- Sometimes a quick check of the patient's story takes place (nurses check their understanding of why the patient is there).
- The nurses usually explain what they are doing when they take observations, or why (for example) they must change patients into gowns.
- Most often they announce the (pending) arrival of the doctor.

---

[1] Based on Martin (1992) and Eggins and Slade (1997/2006), for casual conversation and adapted for healthcare contexts by Jeannette McGregor as part of the project *Emergency communication: addressing the challenges in healthcare discourses and practices.*

In the nursing admission stage, important aspects of communication are those that recognise the patient's transition to the institutional setting of the emergency department, and to try to allay fears about illness or injury. Ways to do this include providing supportive and reassuring feedback, responding to a patient's anxiety about their medical condition, developing shared knowledge and explaining the processes of what is happening and what will happen next.

3.4   Medical Consultations

The initial and final medical consultations constitute the last two activity stages of a typical patient's journey throughout the emergency department. These consultations are separated from each other by the need for patients to undergo tests and wait for the results to come through. In the first medical consultation, doctors will explore the patient's condition, take their history, and then formulate test plans. After the test results come through, a final medical consultation will take place, and will largely be characterised by the delivery of a patient's diagnosis, treatment and disposition.

We examined the internal structure of the medical consultations of 82 patients, in order to establish whether we could discern a generalisable structure across the two activity stages of the medical consultations. Our analysis revealed that clinicians generally talk through a predictable sequence of steps or stages when they perform these medical consultations. We will refer to this predictable structure as generic stages (Hasan 1985; Eggins and Slade 1997/2006). Each stage fulfils a different function in the overall goal of the medical consultation, and we can identify predictable language and vocabulary features in each stage. We can recognise the stages of a medical consultation as having particular functions because of the patterning of communication in each stage. The generic stages are:

(Greeting) $^\wedge$ Initial contact $^\wedge$ Exploration of condition^n History-taking^n Physical examination $^\wedge$ (Diagnostic tests/procedures)^n Consultation with other doctors $^\wedge$ Diagnosis $^\wedge$ Treatment $^\wedge$ Disposition $^\wedge$ (Goodbyes) (Slade et al. 2008)[2]

Although individual variations in the sequence occur because of interruptions or the sheer complexity of the emergency department environment, these are usually minor. For example, in the medical consultations of one emergency department patient, David (who presented with swollen testes), the pattern of clinician–patient turns of talk proceeded sequentially as follows:

- Greeting {turn 1–3}
- Exploration of condition/history-taking {turn 4–67}
- Examination {turn 68–116}
- Diagnosis {turn 117–136}
- Treatment {turn 137–183}, including testing {turn 164–169}
- Disposition {turn 184–188}
- Goodbyes {turn 189–190}.

---

[2] The caret sign $^\wedge$ means that the stage to the left precedes the one to the right. The stages within the brackets () are optional features of the genre; n indicates that a stage is recursive.

Although the generic structure is presented in a linear fashion (above) and is similar to general practice doctor–patient consultations, what makes it different in the emergency department context is its repetitiveness and nonlinear realisation. Some generic stages, such as *exploration of condition*, can occur again and again across the medical consultations. In some cases, the patient may be required to see a specialist, who may repeat the *exploration of condition* for a third time. This recursive process is a regular practice in tertiary emergency departments, where senior clinicians often retake patient narratives that were initially elicited by junior clinicians. In some cases, more senior consultants also revisit the presenting conditions to confirm that patients should be admitted to their clinical team within the hospital.

This recursive, institutional practice is a risk management mechanism, which allows for checks by a number of increasingly senior and experienced clinicians. It enhances patient safety, because new questioning can reconfirm previously proffered diagnoses, and/or it can also allow for untainted exploration as information is heard, and therefore checked, anew. However, as patients are very rarely informed about the processes they will go through in the emergency department or why they will see many different clinicians, this repetition can be frustrating. It can increase anxiety, rather than help alleviate it, especially for those from a language background other than English. We can reasonably assume that most patients would not be as familiar with the emergency consultation context as with the more predictable consultation exchanges conducted during a visit to a general practitioner (GP). The repetition of these stages, first by a junior doctor and then a little later in the consultation by a senior doctor, is demonstrated in the junior/senior extracts presented below.

Many patients we observed or recorded were also confused by the constant interruptions that can occur at any time in an emergency department. Doctors, particularly senior doctors, are frequently interrupted and called away from a consultation to attend to another matter. When they return, they often do not return to the same stage that they left. The patient remembers where they were up, to but the doctor comes in and starts somewhere else.

Our analysis of the emergency department data revealed that clinicians and patients often have different goals during consultations (cf. Gu 1996), though they share the general aim of making a patient well as soon as possible. Clinicians want information to make a diagnosis as soon as possible, while patients often want to tell their story. Patients in the study sometimes received mixed messages when they were asked by doctors to tell their story at the beginning of a consultation, using strategies such as 'Tell me what happened yesterday', interspersed with information-seeking questions.

The 'tell me' request could evoke a simple record of a sequence of events, but we found that what the doctors wanted was a narrative—something with more of a story structure. That is, they wanted patients to give a detailed description of what happened in relation to their visit to the emergency department in a narrative structure sequence with an orientation (beginning), complication, evaluation and ending (see, Labov and Waletzky 1997; Eggins and Slade 1997/2006). In other words, the clinicians are interested in an orientation ^ complication sequence. During the exploration of condition and history-taking stages, doctors gathered information about the patient's pressing concern (such as pain, bleeding, vomiting or a rash) and there then seemed to be an assumption on the part of the doctors that a complication or a particular event had precipitated the emergency department visit (for example, 'Then X happened', 'Then I felt Y'). Our analysis showed that patients generally like to be asked their story. However, their narratives often produced several complications, and these were found to occur in various places within the narrative. Our data also showed that patients' narratives were often interrupted by clinicians asking further questions, which took the narrative in another direction, or moved the consultation to a specific information-seeking question–answer sequence. Thus the stories became fragmented and focus on the complications was lost. This meant that sometimes clinicians failed to pick up on key information, and diagnosis was delayed.

3.4.1   Comparative Effectiveness of the Communication Styles of Senior and Junior Doctors

Seniority emerged as an important communication variable in the medical consultations. Our data indicates that junior and senior doctors display different patterns of talk in their interactions with patients. For example, junior doctors are normally responsible for the exploration of condition and history-taking stages. Junior doctors are often so focused on performing this challenging and difficult task that they concentrate on medical aspects and do not always develop an effective interpersonal relationship with the patient. One senior doctor told us that junior doctors avoid getting involved personally in case patients want medical information that the junior doctors feel too inexperienced to provide. By contrast, in the final three stages of diagnosis, treatment and disposition, senior doctors are more likely to attend to the interpersonal needs of the patient and to negotiate compliance with treatment.

Junior doctors are still learning about their situational practice and of course they vary in experience, training and clinical skills as well as in cultural approaches, all of which can affect care, as the example of patient 37, Nola (PR bleeding), indicates.

The following examples are taken at different times in the consultation. In the consultation, Nola has two rectal examinations, the first conducted by the junior doctor, the second conducted by the gastroenterology registrar. Nola was very embarrassed about the rectal examination she had undergone earlier at the GPs, relaying how she had reacted when her GP said he wanted to examine her in his rooms, to which she had exclaimed 'Here and now?'

When the junior doctor then said 'I'*m going to have to do an examination of your bottom. OK*'? she replied 'That's gonna be horrible… '. She was also embarrassed about the pad she was wearing for the bleeding, and concerned about unhooking the drip that was attached to her. Both doctors use a comfort statement about the drip before the examination: the junior doctor says 'That's OK'; the senior doctor says '*Yeah, the drip'll be alright*'. Below we see the language differences in the way the two doctors went about the examination.

More effective: senior doctor	Less effective: junior doctor
Doctor: Could I get you to roll on to your side? Patient: Yeah, but what about the things, are they OK? These. Doctor: The drip? Patient: Yeah Doctor: Yeah, the drip'll be alright Patient: OK Patient: I've got a … Doctor: That's it Patient: Now, I've got this horrible old pad still on from this morning Doctor: Don't you worry about that. I'm just going to have a bit of a–sneak a bit of a look around it, OK? Patient: OK Doctor: That's it. Roll over. Good-oh. Anyone in your family had bowel cancer at all Mrs [patient's surname]? Patient: No Doctor: Have you lost any weight recently? Patient: No Doctor: Oopsy-daisy. Just see if you can roll right on over. That's the way. Had any trouble with tummy pains recently? Patient: No Doctor: Just relax, I'm going to have a little feel Patient: Right Doctor: All done	Doctor: Just gonna pop the bed down Patient: Now, what's gonna happen? Doctor: (), So what I'll get you to do is to roll over on to your side Patient: Ooh, what about this? Is that OK? Doctor: That's OK. Yep, just shuffle across and tilt towards me. That's right Patient: (). [Background noise, Distant from mic] Doctor: OK Doctor: Now can you bring your knees up? Bend your knees up for me. Do you think you could do that? Patient: Yes, how's that one. Oh excuse me, Doctor (.) [distant from mic] Doctor: It's alright [background noise and voices] Doctor: I'll just pop your pants down Patient: [patient groans] Doctor: Now first of all I'm just going to have a look at the outside of your bottom, OK? Doctor: Right Doctor: I'm just going to pop one finger into your bottom, OK? [patient groaning] Doctor: That's it all over. (). [distant from mic] Patient: Pull up my pants ()
In this example, the senior doctor has a very different approach to Nola's rectal examination than the junior doctor's alongside. He is not as explicit about the step-by-step process and this may be less confronting. He also combines the examination with taking a history; he does not spell out the procedure; he uses more fluent procedural language, which accompanies his actions. He uses everyday colloquial language such as 'sneak a bit of a look' (as opposed to 'I'm just going to put my finger up your bottom') and 'Oopsy daisy', 'Good-oh' and 'Just relax, I'm going to have a little feel'. In the senior doctor's examination, Nola, who has also been schooled by the earlier examination, does not display her embarrassment or discomfort once. The senior uses more instructive language than the junior doctor: 'Don't you worry about that' and 'Roll over'	In this example, the junior doctor uses very procedural language e.g. 'Can you bring your knees up? … I'll just pop your pants down' and so on. The junior doctor follows what they are taught to do, the protocol, which is to explain and spell out each step of the examination process. This makes the procedure somewhat laboured and maybe even a little more daunting. On a number of occasions Nola is heard to groan during the examination. She was discomforted and embarrassed. Although the junior doctor instructs the patient early on 'Yep, just shuffle across and tilt towards me', she subsequently asks Nola gently to comply: 'Now can you bring your knees up? Bend your knees up for me. Do you think you could do that'?

3.4.2   Initial Medical Consultation: Greeting, Initial Contact, Exploration of Condition, History-Taking, Diagnostic Tests and Procedures

In Australia, other than for critical cases the initial medical consultation will generally be conducted by a junior doctor, under the broader supervision of a senior medical colleague. The main focus for the doctor in this stage will be on taking the patient's history and conducting an initial physical examination. The doctor may also order tests (blood tests, CT/X-ray scans, etc.), establish an initial diagnosis (or hypothesis) and initiate treatment, if required.

Although this stage is characteristically dominated by the doctor–patient interview, nurses will often be present at the patient's bedside, providing more evidence of the multidisciplinary nature of emergency department care. While some low-level interventions are carried out, nursing staff will constantly monitor patients, checking whether patients are stable and comfortable. In 'fast track', senior nurses may conduct an initial history and instigate certain tests and treatment before the doctor's appearance at the patient's bedside.

As this stage follows admission, by the time of the first medical consultation, each patient will already have been allocated a bed. The patient's bed is surrounded by curtains, sometimes closed when doctors examine or treat patients to provide visual (not aural) privacy, but generally left open. There are usually comfortable spaces between each bed, with very little furniture apart from the beds and an occasional chair. Most medical equipment is mounted on the wall behind the beds. Some patients sleep, some talk to clinicians or family members, others watch. The activity and noise of the emergency department go on around them.

Observation Field Notes in Subacute Area, 6 pm

Six people are present on the 'station': one nurse, five doctors, two on the phone. There is a lot of noise coming from the X-ray area, separated from subacute only by a cotton curtain. A doctor knocks on examination room 1, and says 'Oh, sorry. I was just looking for Dr X'. He closes the door. Another doctor is on the phone. A nurse is standing by. Another doctor is unpacking some equipment (saline drip) and she then goes into room 4. There is the sound of someone coughing. Someone's buzzer keeps going off. Someone is typing on a computer. Another doctor takes a call. There is the sound of a blood pressure trolley being pushed down the corridor. The phone rings. It is answered by a nurse, 'Yep, thanks so much'.

In most acute sections of the emergency department, cubicles (each defined by curtains) line a number of sides of the room. Doctors, nurses, wardsmen and clerical staff constantly search for people, equipment and information:

Nurse: Has anyone seen the ultrasound machine?
Doctor: Where has patient 10 gone?
Doctor: Are you OK? [doctor to patient walking down corridor]
Doctor: Do you know where you're going? [doctor to patient as patient enters the emergency department doors]
Doctor: Somebody ought to answer that phone. Where is our Katie? [clerical assistant]
Nurse: Did you do an Admission for X?
Wardsman: I've come to collect patient 11. Does anyone know where he's gone?
CC: Has anyone taken the notes I left here?
Doctor: Now where's Simona? Have you seen Simona? She had an elbow she wanted me to look at.

Indeed constant activity is the theme of the acute section, as demonstrated by this researcher's field notes:

Observation Field Notes in Acute, One Morning, 11 am

11.15 am—A patient in EMU rustles a tobacco pouch. Voices can be heard. Three beepers go off. A nurse goes to bed 10, she then looks at the 'station' and speaking loudly says 'We are just going to move you. Just around the corner.' A patient coughs. Two nurses go past. A mental health nurse goes past. He talks to the patient at bed 10. A nurse opens a drawer. Two nurses walk past again. One nurse keeps walking past with a glass of water. The doctor talks to the patient in bed 10. One nurse goes past. The cleaner sweeps the floor.

11.20 am—A doctor is at the side of 'station' with gloves. The cleaner sweeps the floor. The doctor at the 'station' is organising tests. Two wardsmen plus the radiographer bring back the patient from bed 8. Silently. The cleaner is sweeping. There is a carer at the end of bed 9. The cleaner is sweeping. The doctor washes her hands. A woman talks to the patient in bed 8. A patient coughs. A patient goes past bed 10. Two beepers go off. A nurse says to a patient, 'So Mr X tell me why you came in today.' A doctor walks past. A doctor comes off the 'station' and the level of voices rises. A doctor says to the patient in bed 12, 'I'm one of the doctors. Which medication are you taking? Is it the tablet or the injection? But this bottle is very old. Is this from last year? How many did you take? When?' '5 pm' 'You told the nurse midnight. You took 80. You told the nurse 50.' The level of voices is rising. Two doctors come off the 'station'.

11.25 am—The nursing unit coordinator walks past. A patient walks past. Two doctors go past, talking to each other. Bed 10 curtains are opened. Two nurses are talking to each other. Then they talk to the doctor. A senior doctor is helping other doctors doing exams. 'Apparently pharmacy rang and said the dose was too high for her weight.' A wardsman goes past with someone. A doctor talks to the nurse at the end of bed 8. He gives a verbal instruction. The doctor asks about the patient in bed 8. 'If she's had breakfast at all. If she's diabetic she will have to eat something'.

The 'fast track' sections of some emergency departments have a number of consultation rooms where patients are seen. There are also plaster rooms, procedure rooms, and eye and ear, nose and throat rooms so that treatment procedures can be done on the spot.

3.4.3 Communication in the Initial Medical Consultation

This is the stage when the patient will first interact with their doctor, and thus it is when patients will be asked to articulate the nature of their symptoms and concerns, and the doctor will draw on this to plan further tests and hypothesise a diagnosis. Asking and answering questions is one of the principal ways in which doctors and patients will communicate. Doctors will use questions to uncover the medical aspects of the patient's condition, while the patient's main contribution will be to provide information in response. Although meanings are co-constructed through this question and answer process, we observed that doctors clearly dominated the talk and set the agenda for the consultations.

The kinds of questions asked vary according to the type of information doctors want. Questions can be used to encourage patients to contribute relevant information and become collaborators in their diagnosis and treatment, perhaps through asking questions of their own. Alternatively, clinicians' use of questions can position patients as passive 'co-agents', whose only role is to respond as briefly as possible to the clinicians' requests for information. Because time, space and medical expertise are often limited, patients are often positioned as passive in the history-taking process and are not always given the opportunity to offer an opinion, or to ask questions about their own medical condition.

The gravity of the responsibility for the medical outcomes of the consultation appeared to constrain more junior doctors from engaging with patients at an informal level to some extent. We observed that these doctors tended to maintain a greater professional distance from patients than nurses, evident in their choice of words and the degree to which they responded to patients on a personal level. This means that in the interactions between doctor and patient, interpersonal communication was often not a priority. Our data also showed that patients were more likely to respond to nurses in an informal way, and they asked nurses for explanations more often than they asked doctors. We acknowledge that traditional attitudes to the perceived differences between the nursing and medical professions in terms of social hierarchy do play a role in the way patients behave with clinicians. This is particularly the case with elderly patients, many of whom have been conditioned to believe that it is not appropriate to question the doctor.

A registrar we interviewed described the importance of keeping the patient informed about what is going on throughout this stage, particularly when patients were left to wait for test results and might not be seen again by their doctor for an extended period of time. Junior doctors are unable to make final decisions about a diagnosis or an ongoing management/treatment plan in the emergency department. This can mean that there is a delay while a more senior doctor or a specialist is contacted. From the patient's point of view, a clear explanation about what is going to happen next can make a difference. Nurses were frequently relied on by their medical colleagues to 'fill the gaps', keeping patients updated on the process of their care, particularly when doctors would be pulled away to attend other patients:

> Well, 'cause what I do is when I see them initially and then examine [them]—do a history and then examine them, I have some sort of an idea of what's going on and right there and then I explain to them already what I'm thinking, what I'm going to do because it may take a while before I come back to them and review them. Because it takes a while for the bloods to come out, the results of the X-rays and … I don't want them to be in a loss. So it's very important that even during that very first time that I see them, I let them know that it's going to be a wait. 'Cause they would also see me to—doing other things and other patients and all that. And most of the time that's a complaint that … 'Oh the doctor saw me' but then 'I don't know what's going to happen or anything', you know? There would be lots of times when you wouldn't be able to get back to them right away because you're trying to sort out other patients or a new patient comes in and all that. So it's good if your nurses would be able to let them know that yeah, 'We're just waiting for the results' and help you also explain to the patients about what's going on in that time. (Registrar)

A 'move analysis' of the spoken contributions of doctors, nurses and patients in this activity stage (across recorded data) confirmed the communication roles of nurses in providing more explanations to patients about the emergency department processes in this stage. While doctors' interactions with patients were dominated by questions designed to achieve an accurate medical history and exploration of the patient's presenting condition, the nurses' interactions were dominated by statements to keep patients informed about what was happening to them and what they were waiting for. Overall, the doctor's principal communicative role in relation to the patient in the emergency department is one of enquiry, while that of the nurses is to provide information and explanation. Patients were more likely to provide information than to ask questions, both in response to clinicians' questions and when adding information of their own about their medical condition and their experiences through the medical system. They asked relatively few questions.

3.4.4 Summary: Communication in the Initial Medical Consultation

- Doctors' questions dominate this stage, focusing mainly on the patient's illness/injury.
- Nurses ask questions to establish that patients are stable and pain-free.
- Patients mostly respond to doctors' questions. In most cases (but not all) they ask few questions themselves.
- Patients rarely ask questions about what is going to happen to them while they are in the emergency department.
- Doctors' statements are more focused on providing information about the hospital system.
- Nurses provide information to patients about the hospital system and explain what is happening to them, and what their medical condition *means* in terms of consequences or treatment.

The information patients receive is generally limited to what they can expect to happen up until the end of this particular activity stage.

This is the stage in which doctors and nurses have the best opportunity to develop an interpersonal relationship with the patient, as this is the longest stage of the consultation. Unfortunately, it is mostly junior doctors who have carriage of this stage, and they struggle under both the disciplinary and communicative weight of the initial history-taking.

The important aspects of language and communication in the initial medical consultation are those that maximise the exchange of information between the clinicians and the patient about the patient's illness and/or injury, and those that establish trust. These include clinicians greeting patients and introducing themselves and their roles, finding out what the patient already knows, allowing the patient to tell their story, and valuing issues that are important to the patient. If treatment is commenced, it would also be important for clinicians to negotiate treatment and explain the reasoning processes for testing and treatment.

3.4.5   Final Medical Consultation: Diagnosis, Treatment and Disposition

This is the final stage of a patient's emergency department care. It is when patients will have their diagnosis confirmed and decisions will be made about their treatment and disposition (whether the patient should be admitted to a ward or can go home). What happens and who is involved in this final stage differs in the following ways from the initial medical consultation outlined above.

Firstly, in this stage patients will generally first meet the senior doctors who will supervise their care. Sometimes junior and senior doctors attend the bedside together. Senior doctors may use the final history-taking as a teaching opportunity for their more junior counterparts. They may ask them for their opinions to see what they are thinking: Doctor 2: 'OK. So after talking to her, what do you think? Vertigo or pre-sync'? Doctor 1: 'Um—it sounds a bit more like vertigo'. Doctor 2: 'No, I don't think so. I think it's presyncope.' Alternatively, senior doctors may just have junior doctors there to observe, as part of their situational training.

Secondly, the final medical consultation is geared towards preparing for the patient's departure from the emergency department. The patient will be provided with documentation, aimed at securing continuity of care. If a patient is going to a ward, all their notes, X-rays and other test results are gathered on the bed. In the background, generally beyond the patient's earshot, senior doctors will negotiate with inpatient teams in the wider hospital to clear the patient's transfer from the emergency department to another ward for further treatment and supervision. If a patient is going home, after their diagnosis doctors bring final letters of recommendation for the patients' GPs or specialists and talk to patients about treatment plans and follow-up regimes. If patients need to be assessed for special care after they leave the hospital, the Agedcare Services Emergency Team (ASET) and acute and post-acute care (APAC) nurses also see the patients now to check home living arrangements. Sometimes going home is not a straightforward matter, as the case of Bertha demonstrates:

Observation Field Notes, Emergency Department Corridor 2.30 pm

Bertha's knee had given way while shopping. She arrived by ambulance. From the ambulance bay, the nurse educator watching her from behind the window said 'She's been shopping in Westfields and she's fallen over.' This was 100 % accurate. After checking Bertha's knee, the doctor told Bertha there was nothing wrong and she could go home. However Bertha was unable to walk without her walker (which had been taken home in the interim). Bertha could not get a taxi home as she needed support to walk at the other end. Bertha was then assessed by ASET[3] as well as the physio to check her mobility.

Her mobility was not an issue; the lack of her walker was. The hospital was unable to lend her a walker. Hospital records state Bertha left the ED at 13.45 pm, but in fact she sat in the corridor with the researcher from 13.45 pm until 14.30 pm. In that time, the researcher took her to the toilet twice. After the researcher spoke to one of the staff about the fact that she couldn't move from the corridor without assistance, they rang Bertha's neighbour and the neighbour and the neighbour's daughter offered to come and get her and bring the walker with them. Bertha left with them at 14.30 pm.

3.4.6   Communication in the Final Medical Consultation Stage

This final stage follows the same broad clinical process and communication patterns as the initial medical consultation but there is a crucial difference: the final medical consultation is usually the primary responsibility of a senior doctor, who can make conclusive decisions about the diagnosis and patient disposition. The senior doctor takes another patient history, albeit a shorter, more concise version, and will generally deliver a final diagnosis, advise patients on whether they will be discharged home or admitted to a ward in this or another hospital, and in the former case recommend follow-up treatment regimes for patients post-discharge.

The delivery of diagnoses is the key moment of the final medical consultation. It takes significant hospital, clinician and patient effort to reach it safely, accurately and expeditiously. It is what the patient has been waiting for, often very anxiously, and it is what the clinical team assigned to the patient has been working towards. How diagnoses are delivered constitutes a significant communicative event in the patient's journey through the emergency department. The extract below is one example of how this is done. The doctor explains to the patient, Ghadeen, what

---

[3] An ASET nurse is part of the aged-care services in an emergency team.

has happened and what is required for treatment of her sore back. The doctor also checks whether the patient has understood:

Doctor: OK. Good, alright. So your bad news… or y'need good news?
Patient: Have you good news?
Doctor: The good news. Alright. The good news is I…the area where you're sore … is because of not much of padding. Not much of fat tissue over there. When you fell down onto that bone, it's called a coccyx point, the coccyx … bone. It's a very thin area … and when you fell down on to there … it's going to be sore … but most likely you don't need to do anything for it so surgical, surgery-wise or anything like that. That needs to take time… to get better. The bruising is going to be … the … the pain itself … probably at least for one … one week. Do you get me there?

Some doctors make their reasoning processes available to the patient. By including patients in this way, doctors can provide patients with crucial knowledge, which gives them the opportunity of participating in the decision-making process. In the next extract from Estella's consultation (patient 51, spiral leg fracture), the doctor explained very clearly what he could see on Estella's X-ray and his thinking on various options. Estella followed very closely what he was saying, agreeing that the doctor's conclusions were in line with what her GP had been thinking. She pre-empted the doctor's view that a full cast wouldn't be of any use, indicating her full understanding of what he was intending to say:

Doctor: Well, ma'am, okay. Madam, I'm just going to explain to you. You can see the fracture clearly = = here.
Patient: = = Yes, I totally can.
Doctor: It—it looks like in a good position from there. I'm going to talk to one of the senior doctors here just to get her opinion. But usually for such kind of fractures, what we do, we put a half cast.
Patient: Yes, this is what my GP thought it would be.
Doctor: Ah, let me have a look at the other leg. Sorry, madam, just to compare. Yeah, this one is a bit swollen. I believe the swelling is related to the fracture.
Patient: Yes.
Doctor: Okay.
Patient: Yes.
Doctor: So actually a full cast at the moment …
Patient: Yes.
Doctor: … within a few days this swelling is going to be subsided, – – getting down.
Patient: = = Yes, it will, yes.
Doctor: And the full cast it going to be really loose.
Patient: And that won't be = = any use.
Doctor: = = And it's going to be—it's going to be useless.
Patient: Exactly.
Doctor: So what we do is a half cast, get this swelling subsided.
Patient: Yes.
Doctor: And then give it seven days and then I'm going to give you a referral to the fracture clinic.
Patient: Right.
Doctor: You will need to ring, get an appointment done and come [P Yes]—come the day of the appointment you will be seen by the specialist people, ortho wards, and they—they will get a full cast done and give you the good advice.

Providing explanations of what the diagnosis means to patients in words they can understand is pivotal to securing their comprehension of their condition. But as one senior staff specialist we interviewed commented, patient loads and time pressures frequently meant that while doctors would provide basic diagnostic information, they would frequently not 'give [patients] enough time to absorb' what was said or 'allow them to ask questions', to clarify their understanding.

Following the delivery of diagnosis, doctors will then recommend or negotiate a preferred treatment plan with patients. As Cordella (2004, p. 97) noted, if the patient disagrees with the recommended treatment plan, it is likely that they will attempt to renegotiate or even openly refuse to comply. The language strategies employed by clinicians at this stage are therefore critical if they are to succeed in convincing the patient to follow their recommendations. In the following extract, we see the hospital registrar advising Chaitali about the available treatment options, allowing little room for negotiation and showing little empathy.

> *Doctor: So I'll see you again tomorrow. If the bleeding settles down with the medication we'll leave it as it is. Okay? And we'll let you go. But if the bleeding continues to increase, then we'll consider doing something else. Okay? Really what are the options? Well you really have the definitive option. The definitive option is the radiotherapy.*
> *Patient: Oh my God.*
> *Doctor: Okay?*

Indeed across our data, we had little evidence of patients being given the space to negotiate recommended treatment plans. Many doctors commented in the interviews or during our discussions on the floor that they just did not have time to involve the patients effectively. As we hope to demonstrate in this book it is more reliable and safer in terms of accurate diagnoses and compliance with treatment to involve the patient even if it does seem to take longer. We also suggest that if you take the whole patient journey into account, giving patients space early on does not necessarily translate into more consultation time overall. For example, not hearing what the patient is really anxious about can result in an inaccurate diagnosis. This can then lead to more doctors needing to be involved, requiring more clarifications and possible readmissions. Other possible reasons for the patients not being given space to tell their story or to negotiate their treatment include the patient's lack of familiarity with the consulting doctor, the patient's limited information about his/ her medical condition, and the intimidating nature of the emergency department itself. However, it is vital that the patient be able to debate, to clarify, to discuss their treatment options. Without securing patient agreement, patients will be less likely to adhere to clinician's recommendations once they leave the emergency department, and may subsequently seek further medical advice somewhere else or ultimately return the emergency department later with the same complaint.

3.4.7 Summary: Communication in the Final Medical Consultation

- Senior doctors once again focus on questions about the patient's illness/injury
- Patients mostly respond to doctors' questions and in most cases (but not all) they ask few questions themselves
- Senior doctors' statements are about diagnosis, the outcome for the patient and next steps
- There is often repetition, checking the patient's comprehension of what has been said
- Nurses focus on the system
- Patients do ask questions in this stage if they are unclear about their diagnosis/treatment
- There is little negotiation about treatment/management plans

The important aspects of language and communication in the final medical consultation are those that recognise the patient's need to fully understand diagnosis and recommended treatment regimes following their discharge. These include negotiating treatment, explaining the reasoning process behind treatment and advice to patients, repeating key information, checking patients have understood it and providing clear instructions for medication and other follow-up treatment. It is also important for clinicians to allow room for the patient to seek further information.

3.5 Conclusion

As we have demonstrated in this chapter, from the point of triage until disposition, patient care follows a sequence of activities. The structure of these activities shapes patient–clinician communication throughout the patient journey, and produces predictable patterns in clinician–patient interactions, as clinicians endeavour to achieve the clinical goals of each stage. We have also sought to demonstrate the communication challenges involved in each activity stage. These challenges, if not overcome, can pose significant risks to patient safety and diminish the overall quality of the patient's emergency department experience. In the next chapter, we will explore these risks more fully by examining the details of clinician–patient interaction, and by tracing how misunderstandings or breakdowns in communication can occur.

References

Cordella, M. (2004). *The dynamic consultation: a discourse analytical study of doctor–patient communication.* Amsterdam: John Benjamins.

Eggins, S., & Slade, D. (2006, first published 1997). *Analysing casual conversation.* London: Equinox.

Engerstrom, Y. (2008). *From teams to knots: Activity-theoretical studies of collaboration and learning at work*. Cambridge: Cambridge University Press.

Gu, Y. (1996). Doctor–patient interaction as goal directed discourse. *Journal of Asian Pacific Communication, 7*(3–4), 1–21.

Hasan, R. (1985). *Linguistics, language and verbal art*. Geelong: Deakin University Press.

Labov, W., Waletzky, J. (1997). Narrative analysis: Oral versions of personal experience. *Journal of Narrative & Life History, 7*(1–4), 3–38.

Martin, J. (1992). *English text: System and structure*. Amsterdam: John Benjamins.

Slade, D., Scheeres, H., Manidis, M., Iedema, R., Dunston, R., Stein-Parbury, J., Matthiessen, C., Herke, M., McGregor, J. (2008). Emergency communication: the discursive challenges facing emergency clinicians and patients in hospital emergency departments. *Discourse & Communication, 2*, 271–298. doi:10.1177/1750481308091910.

Chapter 4
Communication Risk in Clinician–Patient Consultations

4.1 Introduction

In Chap. 3 we followed the patient's journey through the emergency department and looked at how the functional goals changed according to each of the emergency department's 'activity stages', and we described the typical communication patterns of each stage.

In this chapter, we start our detailed description of the language used in the interactions, focusing in particular on the medical consultations—the last two activity stages of the patient's journey. Through a detailed description of the actual interactions, we explore how particular ways of communicating with the patient could jeopardise the quality and safety of the patient experience. By showing examples of actual transcripts we demonstrate the link between communication and the quality and safety of the patient experience, by highlighting moments of communicative risk—points in the interactions where misalignment or misunderstandings occur. We have called these moments potential risk points (PRP), and argue that if these accumulate they potentially affect health outcomes, such as understanding diagnoses, compliance with recommended treatment and comprehension of discharge instructions. The two major factors that contributed to the number of PRPs that occurred and the fact that they were overlooked were, firstly, that there were many junior and trainee clinicians with limited experience and secondly, that time and workload pressures were typical of those in emergency departments (EDs) around the world.

In Chaps. 5 and 6, we will continue our detailed description of the communication at each stage. Chapter 5 outlines strategies clinicians can use to communicate medical knowledge and information effectively. Chapter 6 describes interpersonal strategies clinicians can use to effectively involve patients in decisions about their care.

© Springer-Verlag Berlin Heidelberg 2015
D. Slade et al., *Communicating in Hospital Emergency Departments,*
DOI 10.1007/978-3-662-46021-4_4

4.2 Link Between Communication and Health Outcomes

A significant body of research (discussed in the Introduction) has established the link between communication, patient involvement, health outcomes and ultimately patient safety, but establishing a direct link can be problematic, particularly in contexts involving spoken communication. Factors that affect health outcomes include patient satisfaction—such as confidence and trust in clinicians—clinician–patient agreement and shared understanding and patient adherence to clinician-recommended treatment plans. All of these affect both the quality and safety of the patient care. Street et al. (2009) argue that the link between communication and health outcomes is usually indirect:

> In most cases [they write], communication affects health through a more indirect or mediated route through proximal outcomes of the interaction (e.g., satisfaction with care, motivation to adhere, trust in the clinician and system, self-efficacy in self-care, clinician–patient agreement, and shared understanding) that could then affect health or that could contribute to the intermediate outcomes (e.g., adherence, self-management skills, social support) that lead to better health. (Street et al. 2009, p. 297)

The difficulty of establishing a direct link between communication and health outcome can be shown by forensic investigations into critical incidents (avoidable patient harm) in hospitals. Spoken communication failures might be a salient issue, but there is rarely a record of the exact series of communicative problems that led to a critical incident. The investigation often takes place many months after the event, and cannot rely on what was actually said in interactions involving the patient.

In this chapter, we demonstrate that by recording and analysing what was actually said in the interactions, we can locate moments in the interactions where misalignment or misunderstandings occur. By identifying and describing these vulnerable points, we can predict the types of communicative practices that can lead to misalignments which can cumulatively affect the quality and safety of the patient experience. We have coined the term 'potential risk point' to describe the moment in the interaction between clinician and patient when misalignments or misunderstandings take place. Post-event analyses usually indicate that critical incidents are caused by the accumulation of multiple problems, rather than by a single isolated problem.

In this chapter, we provide examples from the audio recordings of potential risk points. The examples show that moments of communicative risk—such as failure to track the patient's narrative, failure to pick up on the patient cues, or inadequately informing the patient—can lead to patient dissatisfaction and lack of agreement and understanding of the treatment plan. This in turn can affect health outcomes and ultimately patient safety.

Street et al. (2009) describing the relationship between communication and health outcomes explains:

> For example, a clinician's clear explanations and expressions of support could lead to greater patient trust and understanding of treatment options (proximal outcomes). This in turn may facilitate patient follow-through with recommended therapy (an intermediate outcome), which in turn improves a particular health outcome (e.g., disease control, emotional well-being). Or, patient participation in the consultation could help the physician better

understand the patient's needs . . . as well as discover possible misconceptions the patient might have about treatment options. (Street et al. 2009, p. 297)

Exploring communicative risk, we argue that the last activity stage of the patient journey—the final medical consultation (which includes diagnosis, treatment and disposition)—is communicatively more vulnerable than other parts of the emergency department consultation. In this stage, misunderstandings or miscommunications have greater potential for adverse consequences for the patient than if breakdowns occur during other times in the consultation.

Focusing on the final medical consultation—diagnosis, treatment and disposition—we analyse a number of misunderstandings or miscommunications—the potential risk points. By analysing the different ways in which clinicians and patients respond to potential risk points, we show how specific language or communication strategies can lead to negative health outcomes.

In the last section of the chapter, we propose a 'systemic order of risk' which distinguishes communicative risk from other kinds or risk such as social or biomedical risks.

4.3 Potential Risk Points in the Consultation

In Chap. 3, we described the overall structure of the initial and final medical consultations (the final two activity stages), outlining the predictable sequence that consultations go through. By examining many instances of emergency department interactions, we were able to determine how the medical consultations are normally structured into predictable stages, each stage having its own choices in meaning, reflected in characteristic patterns of wording.

Of the stages we identified in Chap. 3, our analysis suggests some have a higher potential risk than others. In particular, in the initial medical consultation, the *exploration of condition* is a potentially risky moment. Similarly, in the final medical consultation *diagnosis* and *treatment* are the risky moments. These are identified as critical points in the consultation because of their key functions within the medical consultations. It is the primary function of the *exploration of condition* to obtain the exact nature, time frame and pattern of symptoms with which the patient presents. If a clinician fails to track details in the patient's narrative or misses information here, that clinician's differential diagnosis can change significantly. In our analyses below we examine a number of instances where the exchange of information in this stage of the consultation results in potential risk points for the patient.

We also identify the *diagnosis* and *treatment* in the consultation as communicatively critical in terms of potential risk. These are the main points at which clinicians hand over information to the patient about their condition and about follow-up care.

Focusing on potential communication errors in these stages we will now demonstrate the different ways that clinicians and patients respond to potential risk points in the emergency department consultations. Initially, we focus on potential risk points that increase the risks to patient safety. We then examine how risk is either averted or precipitated by clinicians and patients (or relatives) within these stages.

4.3.1   Potential Risk Point: Failure to Track the Patient's Narrative and Listen to the Patient's Cues

In many of the consultations, we identified divergent trajectories between a doctor's line of questioning and the patient's desire to foreground other information, from the intensity of pain they are feeling, to various details surrounding their illness or complaint. Sometimes the doctors did not pick up on the patient cues because they focused solely on the medical diagnosis.

The first examples highlight a number of potential risk points that occur when there is rote questioning and a failure to track the patient's narrative in *exploration of condition.*

The following extract is part of an exchange between a male junior clinician and the patient we call Fahime. The patient is a middle-aged Middle Eastern woman with advanced level English who understands most of the interaction. Fahime's daughter, aged about 20, is fluent in English and translates some of the questions. Two junior clinicians first interview the patient and then a senior female doctor interviews her 54 min after her arrival in the emergency department. She spends 1.5 hrs in the emergency department, of which 51 min are with clinicians. She is eventually diagnosed with emotional distress and depression, after being seen by three different doctors.

Fahime had come to the emergency department suffering dizziness and in a quite severely distressed state. A potential risk point occurs early in this consultation, during the initial *exploration of condition* stage when Fahime tries indirectly to explain the real reason for her attendance at the emergency department: 'And I found my son sick.' It was established later that her son had attempted suicide earlier on the same day, and was in fact still in the same emergency department. But because the patient cues were not picked up on, this was not elicited by any of the clinicians. The junior clinician chooses not to follow up the patient's cue until several minutes later, when he asks, 'And is—what's wrong with your son?' The following interaction then takes place:

Doctor: And is—what's wrong with your son?
Daughter: He's just stressed he's and ==
Doctor: == OK ==
Daughter: == And the situation was inflamed and she became stressed because of that, and it added == to her.
Doctor: == Sure.
Daughter: Yeah.
Doctor: OK. OK.
Doctor: Have you been eating and drinking sort of reasonably normally?
Fahime: I drink but I haven't been eating. ==
Daughter: == She hasn't been eating well because she's just had a recent death in the family. ==
Doctor: OK ==
Daughter: == A couple of days ago. ==

Doctor: OK ==
Daughter: == Which is her grandmamma. ==
Doctor: == OK ==
*Daughter: == So she's been spending a lot of time at her mother's house. And no
    she hasn't been eating well, obviously distressed because of that.*
Doctor: OK. Sure, but you've been keeping up your fluids and drinking and ==

In this extract we see the junior clinician attempting to explore the issue around the
health of the patient's son, but the patient's daughter answers for her mother and
thereby thwarts the flow of the narrative. The daughter's intervention withholds
this key information from the clinician, although it is possibly the very reason for
the patient's presentation on the day. If the daughter had not intervened when she
said 'He's just stressed he's and ===', the junior clinician, and hence the entire
exploration of condition and *history-taking* might have proceeded differently. What
is significant from the patient safety perspective, and insightful in terms of novice
to expert development, is the ease with which the junior clinician is intercepted and
waylaid by the patient's relative.

Later in the *exploration of condition* stage, a second potential risk point occurs
when the patient's daughter tries to explain the reason for her mother not eating well
lately by informing the junior doctor that there had been a recent death in the family. The junior clinician apparently does not register this information as significant
to the presentation of the patient. It is clear the patient is not heard; and we see the
junior clinician attempting to reduce the problem to a biomedical issue.

Figure 4.1 shows the different contributions made by doctors and Fahime and her
family while in the emergency department. The figure shows the striking difference
between questions asked (149 by doctors; 4 by Fahime and her family) and answers
given (141 by Fahime and family; 8 by doctors).

It is reasonable to expect that in the initial history-taking stage the junior doctors might ask many questions and make few statements about the patient's illness.
However, this same pattern continued throughout Fahime's stay in the emergency
department. In addition, most of the questions asked by the doctors across the consultations were closed (yes/no) questions. There were very few open questions (e.g.
'How often do you get dizzy like this?'), which would have given the patient more
scope to expand on her information.

Our analysis of the interactions with Fahime shows that at no stage did the patient get the opportunity to tell her story. As a result, the *real* reason why Fahime
was in the emergency department was not diagnosed until the last senior doctor
came in. She was finally diagnosed with depression and advised to see her general
practitioner (GP). This analysis suggests that either the patient did not feel that it
was appropriate for her to ask questions or she felt too intimidated by the context
to do so.

A number of key points arise from this extract, particularly the in situ complexity
of managing (or even recognising) communicative risk. On the one hand, the senior
doctor who came in later to yet again re-question the patient established that the
patient was distressed. This doctor's diagnosis at that point maximised risk control

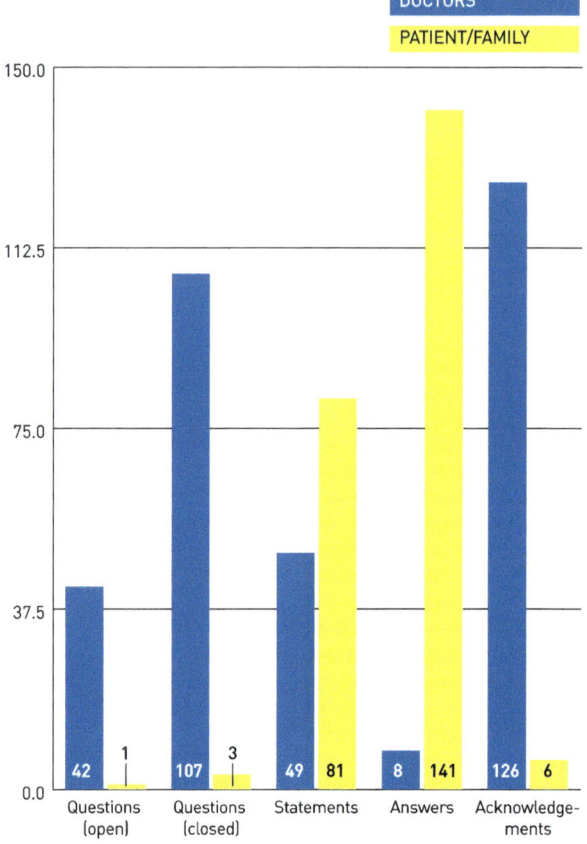

Fig. 4.1 Analysis of questions and statements in the Fahime interaction

as she recognised what was wrong with the patient. This repetition of questions, while providing the safety net of the more senior doctor's expert knowledge, meant submitting an emotionally distressed patient to repeated questioning and diagnostic delay—either or both of which could have led to a deterioration of the patient's emotional state, and to increasing confusion. In a teaching hospital, junior doctors are given the opportunity to conduct *exploration of condition* and *history-taking,* hence there will be times when patients will be exposed to less than satisfactory interviews and contradictory and competing practices. However, this is a case where closer supervision of a junior doctor by a more senior, more experienced clinician in the initial stages of the interview would have been appropriate. The senior doctor on diagnosing the patient with depression advised her that she should see her GP and did recommend treatment. Fahime left anxious and stated to the researcher that she was not satisfied with her treatment.

4.3.2   Potential Risk Point: Patient Involvement—Not Listening to the Patient

Patients occasionally identify potential risk points themselves, and intervene in the interview process as a way of maintaining their own safety. This is clear from the consultation with Zahara, a middle-aged Yugoslavian-born woman but now a fluent English speaker, who presents with severe stomach pain following a surgical abdominal procedure. She had a gastric band inserted some years ago and presented with pain due to suspected slippage of gastric band.

In this consultation a potential risk point occurs during the *treatment* stage, when the junior doctor offers the patient some stronger pain relief ('Do you want to try some Panadeine Forte?'). The patient had already told the doctor that she was allergic to codeine, but the doctor had forgotten this piece of information:

Doctor: Um, and any allergies to any medications?
Zahara: Um nuro—not nurofen, codeine.
Doctor: Codeine?
Later in the consultation
Doctor: Do you want to try some Panadeine Forte?
Zahara: Am I allowed to?
Doctor: Hmmm hmm.
Zahara: Panadeine Forte. Has that got codeine in it?
Doctor: Yes. Oh I'm sorry.
Zahara: ( )
Doctor: ( ) your allergies.

When the doctor offers Panadeine Forte, the patient has a choice of challenging the doctor or of trusting the doctor's judgement. Zahara tentatively challenges the doctor's choice ('Am I allowed to?'). The doctor replies in the affirmative but the patient persists and questions the use of Panadeine. The doctor then suddenly remembers the allergy.

Here we see how the patient herself has avoided a potential risk of an allergic reaction by seeking clarification of the doctor's suggestion. Her involvement is significant, given the unequal power relationship between herself and the clinician. This patient reiterates confusion about processes of the emergency department and the language used by clinicians throughout the consultation:

Doctor: Now you've got some tummy pain following surgery?
Zahara: Uh huh.
Doctor: On Monday is that right?
Zahara: No I didn't have surgery.
Doctor: You had? == Yeah.
Zahara: == I got a lap band. Like, and that was a few years ago but it slipped. I've seen Dr Donovan.
Doctor: Yeah? Yup.
Zahara: And um—he said he wants to replace it with another one.

Doctor: Hm-mm

Zahara: And he said on Monday I had to go and get fluid taken out, all it out to make me comfortable and um, because sometimes there's complications with that that it could have a, a prolapse and that he—'cause I rang them this morning, they're in Melbourne and they said to come straight to St George Hospital 'cause it sounds like a prolapse.

Doctor: OK. So that—

Zahara: == And I've been experiencing it for the past 48 hours.

Doctor: OK and what sort of pain have you been getting?

Zahara: Very, very bad pain right there and I can feel it, you're not supposed to feel the band and I can feel it and I've been vomiting every time I eat and, just extreme pain.

Doctor: Since Monday when you had it done or just == this morning?

In the extract above, Zahara's consultation begins with the junior doctor asking, 'Now you've got some tummy pain following surgery?' using the term 'surgery', which the patient immediately rejects in preference for 'No I didn't have surgery,( ) I got a lap band.' It had been inaccurately recorded in her medical records that she just had the surgery. The doctor's initiating question was based on this inaccuracy, which was not corrected for some time.

These kinds of questions, which Matthiessen (in Slade et al. 2008) refers to as 'assumptive' questions, are prevalent in emergency department consultations where they typically function to check and double-check the doctor's understanding of the patient's responses. However, they can also constrain the responses available to the patient and limit the doctor's expectations, and this can lead to misunderstanding between doctor and patient. This was the case with Zahara, where she was clearly confused about this assumption. Although she tried to correct it, this misunderstanding proceeded for most of the consultation. The way in which the wrong assumption narrowed the doctor's own field of expected response is clearly demonstrated by the way in which he incorrectly interprets even contrary responses to his further assumptions.

Later, after being told that as she is going to be having a computed axial tomography (CAT) scan, and that the doctor would keep her informed, she turns to the researcher and says 'Did you get all that?' At another point after one of the nurses had left, she said 'I heard what she said but I don't know what she said…'—a clear indication of a potential risk point as the patient did not understand the reasons for the procedure or the doctor's explanations.

We have now established that the alignment of clinician and patient understanding and actively listening to the patient is key to minimising patient risk and safety in the emergency department. To be able to assess patient understanding, close tracking of the patient's story by the clinician as well as patient involvement—or agency—in the interaction are essential.

4.3.3   Potential Risk Point: Patient Involvement—Not Informing the Patient

Sometimes communication breaks down and patients are not given critical information regarding their care. Such omissions can trigger sentinel events (US Government Accountability Office GAO 2004) where serious physical risk can result. During our observations in one emergency department, we observed a nurse searching for a patient. She asked her colleagues: 'Has anyone seen the patient from bed 16?' Other staff members asked who the patient was. The patient, who had been involved in an accident, was described as male, with black curly hair, youngish and wearing a neck brace. One of the staff indicated that he had seen this patient walking in the direction of the toilet a short time before. The nurse who was looking for the patient exclaimed: 'But he isn't supposed to be walking around! He hasn't had an X-ray yet!' Another member of staff suggested: 'You should have stuck a sign on him: "This patient should not walk around!"' The patient was located and returned to his bed.

We did not record the outcome of the bed 16 patient's stay in the emergency department, but based on the nurse's level of anxiety about the patient's movements, serious risk to the patient was possible and may have occurred. Through recording, interviews and observations, our study has identified that frequently patients are not informed about what they can or cannot do, or what is about to happen to them. Although this can occur in the high-pressure environment of the emergency department where emergency clinicians struggle to ensure the best possible care under duress, mistakes and omissions are frequently caused by communication breakdowns. From the perspective of patient safety, the two examples above show how listening to patients and adequately informing them at all stages are two important aspects of involving patients in their care, crucially important for minimising risk.

These examples highlight the significant challenges facing both the delivery of emergency medicine and the training of junior clinicians. In a teaching hospital, the training of junior clinicians is central to the work of emergency departments—but some exchanges are risky, as the data above have shown. Yet for clinical experience and learning to be meaningful, this training *ought* to take place in high pressure of the emergency department—a necessity that leaves hospital administrators and medical colleagues, not to mention patients, in potentially precarious circumstances. With the seriously extended and already under-resourced workforce in emergency departments around the world, closer supervision of novices by seniors is difficult, as is the follow-up of their work by senior clinicians, but in many cases it is crucial in terms of both the quality and safety of the patient experience.

4.3.4   Potential Risk Point: Delivery of Diagnosis

The primary tasks of an emergency department clinician are to find out what is wrong with a patient and to work out what the most effective follow-up treatment should be. Thus, diagnoses for all but very minor ailments are usually given to patients after a considerable number of emergency department activities that include several consultations between different clinicians and the patient, one or more physical examinations, tests such as blood tests and X-rays, consultations between junior and senior doctors and, often, telephone consultations with the patient's GP.

The delivery of diagnoses is the key moment of the clinician–patient consultation and one that takes significant hospital, clinician and patient effort to reach safely, accurately and expeditiously. The point at which the diagnosis is delivered during a patient's journey through an emergency department is clearly important. It is what the patient has been waiting for, often very anxiously, and it is what the doctor assigned to the patient has been working towards. The way in which a diagnosis is delivered therefore constitutes a key communicative event in the patient's journey. The interaction below is one example of how a junior doctor (from a non-English speaking background) delivers the news to an elderly male, patient 4 (Clement), who presented with left-sided pain.

Extract 4.4 Patient 4 (Clement)

Doctor: I give you good news or bad news?
Patient: All right.
Doctor: Which one?
Patient: Bad one first.
Doctor: Bad one first. OK we did a scan and we found some clots. Multiple. Several clots in the chest. Right that's the bad news. The good news, we found out why you have clots. It's not from the heart. The heart's not going to fail.
Patient: OK.

The consultations leading up to the delivery of this diagnosis had continued for many hours while lengthy blood and X-ray tests were carried out. The doctor had been extremely busy all day with this patient and others, yet he wanted to finalise the consultation—that is, be the one to tell the patient the diagnosis—before he completed his shift.

In one reading of the exchange, the doctor's language lacks the sensitivity required to convey such critical news to an elderly patient. It could be he realises that the normal biomedical language and interpersonal distance are not quite right in this situation. He picks up on the patient's own earlier use of the *good news, bad news* phrase. This may have been chosen as a deliberate strategy for establishing rapport with the patient, constructing some informality or familiarity, but the patient was left anxious and bewildered.

4.3.5   Communication Breakdowns in Transitions of Care

Lastly, to illustrate organisational difficulties involving communication risk, we present the story of Powell, a 35-year-old male who arrived at the emergency department one day at 3.12 pm. He was triaged at 3.30. He brought with him a letter from his physician addressed to the emergency department director, explaining that he was concerned to make sure the patient was attended to as soon as possible because he had a highly infectious condition—shingles. The letter referred to an earlier conversation between the GP and the emergency department director (at 1.30 pm that day) about the patient. Powell showed the letter to the receptionist and then to the triage nurse.

The triage nurse assigned category 4 to the patient and he was told to wait in the waiting room where a number of other people were waiting, including young children and elderly people. The letter apparently had little effect on the speed with which the patient was attended to.

Powell waited for 2.5 hrs before a nurse suddenly appeared at his side, and began the process of taking him through to the emergency department with some urgency. Because a private interview room was occupied, the patient was asked to wait in the ambulance bay, which was also busy with patients on trolleys waiting to be admitted. Finally, Powell was shown into a room and the nurse began his history-taking and examination. The nurse concluded that the patient did have a highly infectious disease and put a sign on the interview room door advising others not to enter the room. He explained to Powell that his condition was infectious to the elderly, to those with suppressed immune systems and to young children in particular.

The patient, having been made to wait in the waiting room and the ambulance bay for close on 3 hrs that day, had placed a number of people at risk. Neither the receptionist nor the triage nurse reacted to the contents of the letter from the GP regarding the patient's condition. The GP had attempted to pre-empt risk through communicative channels, using both a spoken (phone call) and written (letter) alert. But a number of factors overrode any appropriate medical response and ultimately compromised the safety of several patients within the department.

These are the observation notes taken by our team of researchers on the day:

Powell, a 35-year-old male, was HIV positive. He arrived at the ED one day at 15.12 pm after being diagnosed with severe shingles and being referred there by his GP. Powell was triaged at 15.30 pm and had a letter from his GP addressed to the emergency department director, explaining that Powell had a highly infectious condition—shingles—and should be attended as soon as possible. The letter referred to an earlier conversation between the GP and the emergency department director (at 13.30 pm that day) concerning Powell's forthcoming arrival at the emergency department. Powell showed the letter to both the emergency department receptionist and to the triage nurse.

Powell was triaged as category 4 (although assessed as having a potentially serious condition) and was told to take a seat in the waiting room. At the time there were several other patients in the waiting room, including young children and elderly people. The letter apparently had little effect on the speed with which Powell was attended to, and there was no indication by the triage nurse that sitting with other (sick) people might be a problem. Powell sat in the waiting room for two and a half hours before another nurse approached him. The nurse asked Powell to follow him through the emergency department to the family room where he would perform a rapid assessment of Powell's condition. It transpired however that the family room was already occupied by a patient under police escort. Powell was left to wait in the ambulance bay until the family room became free. The ambulance bay was quite busy with patients on trolleys waiting to be placed in a clinical area of the emergency department. Ten minutes later Powell was shown into the room. After taking his history and conducting a physical exam, the nurse concluded that Powell was indeed suffering from the highly infectious disease shingles. The nurse then put a sign on the interview room door advising others not to enter the room. He explained to Powell that his condition was infectious to the elderly, to those with suppressed immune systems, and to young children in particular.

The fact that Powell had been made to wait in the waiting room and the ambulance bay for almost three hours may have placed a number of people at risk. Neither the receptionist nor the triage nurse had acted upon Powell's letter warning of his infectious condition, possibly because of the high pre-sentation loads and extended waiting times in the emergency department that day. Despite attempts by Powell's GP to pre-empt this risk by both a phone call and a letter, the most appropriate and safest medical response did not eventuate.

Observation field notes: one day in an emergency department waiting room, 12.30 pm

The example of Powell demonstrates how communication can fail between the primary care context and the hospital, demonstrating the challenges and risks in communication that so often occur in the transition of care from the community (e.g. GP) to the hospital or from the hospital back to the community. Poor communication in these transitions has been shown to be a major contributing factor in adverse events, posing direct threats to patient safety (see, for example, Buckley et al. 2013; WHO 2013; Groene et al. 2012; Crane 1997). For example, in Australia, communication errors at discharge are implicated in over 40 % of preventable read-missions to hospital (Muecke et al. 2010).

As reviewed in Chap. 1, much of the research has focused on communication within the hospital up to, and including, the point of discharge. There has been less research on the role of effective communication in the coordination of care between acute and primary care settings, and in the process of achieving seamless continuity of care between these different health care providers. One of the recommendations in Chap. 7 is the pressing need for further research on the role of communication in transitions of care from hospital to the community.

In the next section, we will describe the different kinds of risk that can occur in hospitals and by doing so locating communicative risk on a typology of medical risks.

4.4   Systemic Order of Risk

The type of risk we are concerned with in this book is communicative risk—that is, risk caused by communication gaps, errors or misunderstandings. Communicative risk is of course only one kind of risk that can occur in hospitals; so to finish this chapter we will explore the nature of this type of risk in health care by locating it in an ordered typology of systems in operation in hospitals.

Hospitals are very complex systems, and for patients starting their journeys through an emergency department this complexity can be quite bewildering. However, analytically, we can manage the complexity by deconstructing it into component systems based on an ordered typology of systems (for this ordered typology, see, e.g. Halliday and Matthiessen 2006; Halliday 2005; Matthiessen 2007, 2013[1]). We can then describe the type of risk associated with each system.

There are two broad realms of systems, (1) material systems and (2) immaterial systems:

1. Material systems consist of matter—either inanimate, physical systems, or animate, biological systems. As a set of material systems, a hospital is a building or complex of buildings with medical equipment and other forms of infrastructure; and it is an ecosystem in which biological organisms function in different niches.
2. Immaterial systems are social systems and semiotic (meaning) systems (related to communication, including information flow, in healthcare systems). As a set of immaterial systems, a hospital is a community consisting of people in different roles and in different social groups, including both the professional roles and the roles of patients and other visitors; and these people are constantly exchanging meanings in different communication roles.

A hospital is thus a complex of material and immaterial systems, and can be viewed and analysed physically, biologically, socially and semiotically. This complexity is partly evolved, partly designed—as is typical of complex systems we build such as hospitals, power stations and air traffic control systems. The complexity and risk inheres in each systemic order, but it is, naturally, magnified by the constant interaction between the systemic orders. Van Cott (1994) suggests that healthcare systems are the largest and most complex type, saying (p. 55):

> It ['a healthcare system'] is an enormous number of diverse and semiautonomous elements: ambulance services, emergency care, diagnostic and treatment systems, outpatient clinics, medical devices, home care instruments, patient-monitoring equipment, testing laboratories, and many others. All of these elements are loosely coupled in an intricate network of individuals and teams of people, procedures, regulations, communications, equipment, and devices that function in a variable and uncertain environment with diffused, decentralized management control.

Such systems cannot be allowed to fail, and the fundamental challenge is to design for safe operation with a low degree of risk through robust risk management and

---

[1] This section draws on Matthiessen (2013), and some passages have been included in our discussion.

strategies for error recovery, but this is of course an ideal. Risk is inherent in any designed system; and researchers have compared the operation of different kinds of designed system. For example, the model of crew resource management has been taken from aviation into health care (e.g. Risser et al. 2011; see also Ternov (n.d., 2011)). One general principle is that system designs are faulty if they are based on the mistaken notion that the people involved in the operation of the systems will not make mistakes (cf. Moorman 2007); in other words, systems must be designed to tolerate and cope with mistakes. As we demonstrated with potential (communicative) risk points, most are averted or prevented due to the layers of protection built into the system and it is only when these multiply and cumulate that the patient's safety is at risk.

In health care, there are risks in each of the realms of systems, so there are many kinds of potential errors that need to be reduced. To ensure safer patient care, McClanahan et al. (2011) suggest five key "error reduction strategies":

1. Improve information access
2. Reduce reliance on memory
3. Reduce number of hand-offs (=handovers)
4. Standardize tasks
5. Error-proof processes

On their list, semiotic errors—i.e. errors related to communication in healthcare systems—are absolutely central.

To characterize communicative risk in health care—or semiotic risk—we can locate it in the typology of systems, described above, as in Fig. 4.2.

Errors are risks that have been actualised. Risks may be material in nature (i.e. relating to the world of matter), either physical or biological:

typology of medical risk according to systemic orders

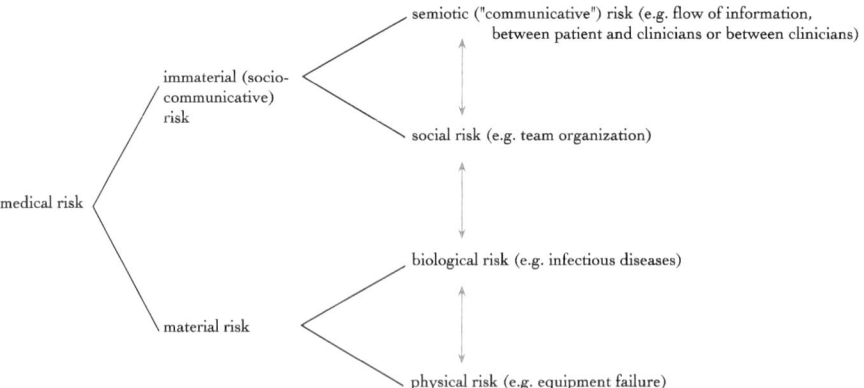

Fig. 4.2 Types of risks in institutions of health care

- In hospitals and other institutions of health care, risks may be physical: Here the risk of failure relates to buildings, equipment—any aspect of the physical infrastructure of an institution of health care; for example, equipment may malfunction.
- Risks may also be biological since institutions of health care are complex ecosystems full of living organisms, including ones that pose a threat because they spread diseases, either bacteria or viruses or hosts to these.

These material risks are potentially life-threatening not only to patients but also to clinicians and other people working in, or visiting, institutions of health care, but they are well-known, and strategies have been developed for dealing with such risks. For example, a century and a half ago, Florence Nightingale pioneered the reduction of biological risk; in her *Notes on Nursing,* she writes that part of the 'very first canon of nursing' is 'to keep the air that [the patient] breathes as pure as the external air'.

Immaterial risks are perhaps even more of a challenge than material ones, partly because they are harder to detect; they are either social or semiotic:

- In hospitals and other institutions of health care, risks may be social: Here the risk of failure relates to the organisation of the hospital, etc., as a social institution—to administration and management, including hierarchies of control, team coordination, bed allocation, patient tracking and all the other myriad of features of professional roles and activities of a modern institution of health care.
- In addition to being social, risks may be semiotic—that is, risks associated with communication. Such risks include the distortion or loss of information in exchanges between patients and clinicians but also between clinicians in clinical handover.

Of these two orders of immaterial risk, communicative risk (semiotic risk) is harder to detect and is less understood. But it is at least as important as material risk, and communication failure can be as life-threatening as material failure. And the different kinds of risks and failures interact. Halliday (2011) comments,

> We see how densely semiotic and material systems interpenetrate if we watch people performing extremely complex tasks. The complexity lies in the subtle and constantly shifting relations between the discourse and its situational context. If we consider the work practices in high risk environments, such as air traffic control rooms, surgical operating theatres or nuclear power stations, the interface between matter and meaning is critical [...] When accidents occur, as they will as predicted by the "Swiss cheese" theory, they have typically been explained as instantial failures [...]

For the Swiss cheese model, see Reason (1990): The holes in a Swiss cheese represent weaknesses in a system, and when the holes align, accidents are very likely to occur—what Reason (1990: Sect. 10.2.5) calls 'a trajectory of accident opportunity'. As Halliday points out, failures are typically treated as one-off failures (i.e. instantial failures) without any attempt to relate them to the system that must have engendered them. Halliday goes on to note that instantial failures must be interpreted systemically, i.e. related to the system that engendered them—which takes us back to failure potential, or risk.

4.5   Communication as a Risk Factor in Patient Safety

Debate persists about the *extent* to which communicative risk contributes to risks to patients' safety. To date, the outcomes of specialised professional practices such as technological and scientific specialisation have been seen as more significant for patient safety than the organisational and communicative dimensions of clinical practice. This is reflected in the World Health Organization (WHO) taxonomy, which lists poor teamwork or inadequate communication as *contributing* factors only. The WHO defines a contributing factor as a 'circumstance, action or influence…which is thought to have played a part in the origin or development of an incident, or to increase the risk of an incident' (WHO 2007), p. 7). In their complex taxonomy they foreground the significance of the relationship of other more technological and scientific practices to patient safety. Others contend, however, that professional practices will only be as good as the organisational and communicative processes that support and facilitate them (see, for example, Kohn et al. 1999; Iedema 2005), the language and structural dimensions of work therefore being as critical to patient safety as biomedical accuracy.

In this chapter, we focused on communicative risk, and identified two stages of a patient's trajectory through the emergency department, *exploration of condition* and *diagnosis/treatment* as more communicatively significant than other stages due to the critical nature of information exchanged between patients and clinicians. We explored the impact of some of the language choices of clinicians in these stages at the very moments they appeared to cause potential risk—at the PRPs—and we started to highlight the links between risks to patient safety and communication. If misunderstanding or miscommunications occurred, these were no longer just 'circumstances, actions or influences' playing a part in the origin of harm, but potentially, they were a central component of it.

We presented a number of exchanges conducted by junior doctors. Those who relied initially on a rote checklist approach for the questioning of patients (as an insurance against missing key aspects of the patient's history) were shown to have been too focused on the sequence of differential diagnostic questioning, and to have missed other cues from patients. In one instance, iatrogenic harm was avoided only when the patient challenged the doctor's advice, based on information she had already given the doctor about her allergies to medication.

4.6   Conclusion

Communicative risk is inevitably pervasive in a hospital and occurs as a result of gaps and misunderstandings in the flow of information from one medical consultation to another, or from one clinician to another, as well as in misunderstandings between patients and clinicians in consultations. While these gaps are not always catastrophic or even problematic (Cook et al. 2000) we must be aware of how, where and when they are the most likely to occur. Viewed from the patient's perspective, these gaps may occur at any point in the consultation, but we noted that in the course of the emergency department journey some stages are more communicatively vulnerable than others, and hence more critical to the patient's safety.

The immense complexity of what emergency clinicians do, and what actually occurs in the multiple interactions with the patients, becomes visible only with actually recording all the interactions the patients have with clinicians during their stay in the emergency department.

We believe that communicative risk management requires a review of organisational processes, current communicative systems—the flow of information and the nature of the interactions that occur—and development of training materials and programs, and the design of computational support systems. However, regardless of which steps are taken, solutions must be built around in-depth analysis of solid evidence emerging from empirical studies of actual communication. Through close analysis of exchanges between clinicians and patients, and among clinicians, we begin to see how communication failures occur and how patients are exposed to risk. It is only through doing this that it will be possible to develop strategies and solutions to address these problems.

References

Buckley, B., McCarthy, D., Forth, V., Tanabe, P., Schmidt, M., Adams, J., Engel, K. (2013). Patient input into the development and enhancement of emergency department discharge instructions: A focus group study. *Journal of Emergency Nursing, 39*(6), 553–561.

Cook, R.I., Render, M., & Woods, D.D. (2000). Gaps in the continuity of care and progress on patient safety. *BMJ (Clinical research ed.), 320,* 791–794.

Crane, J. (1997). Patient comprehension of doctor-patient communication of discharge from the emergency department. *Journal of Emergency Medicine, 15*(1), 1–7.

Groene, R., Orrego, C., Suñol, R., Barach, P., Groene, O. (2012). 'It's like two worlds apart: An analysis of vulnerable patient handover practices at discharge from hospital'. *BMJ Quality & Safety, 21,* i67–i75.

Halliday, M.A.K. (2005). On matter and meaning: The two realms of human experience. *Linguistics and the Human Sciences, 1*(1), 59–82.

Halliday, M.A.K. (2011). Halliday in the 21st century. In J. Webster (Ed.), *The collected works of M.A.K. Halliday* (Vol. 11). London: Continuum.

Halliday, M.A.K., & Matthiessen, C.M.I.M. (2006). Construing experience through meaning: A language-based approach to cognition. Study edition (of #4). London: Continuum.

Iedema, R. (2005). Medicine and health: Intra- and inter-professional communication. In K. Brown (Ed.), *Encyclopaedia of language and linguistics* (pp. 745–751). Oxford: Elsevier.

Kohn, L.T., Corrigan, J.M., & Donaldson, M.S. (1999). *To err is human: Building a safer health system.* Washington DC: National Academy Press.

Matthiessen, C. M.I.M. (2007). The lexicogrammar of emotion and attitude in English. In electronic *Proceedings of the Third International Congress on English Grammar* (ICEG 3), Sona College, Salem, Tamil Nadu, India, January 23-27, 2006.

Matthiessen, C. M.I.M. (2013). Applying systemic functional linguistics in healthcare contexts. *Text and Talk, 3*(4–5), 437–466.

McClanahan, S., Goodwin, S.T., & Perlin, J.B. (2011). A formula for errors: Good people + bad systems. In P. Spath (Ed.), *Error reduction in health care: A systems approach to improving patient safety*. San Francisco: Jossey-Bass.

Moorman, D.W. (2007). Communication, teams, and medical mistakes. *Annals of Surgery, 245*(2), 173.

Muecke, S., Kalucy, E., & McIntyre, E. (2010). 'Continuity and safety in care transitions: Communication at the hospital/community care interface', research roundup Australian primary health care research and information service.

Reason, J. (1990). *Human error*. Cambridge: Cambridge University Press.

Risser, D. T., Simmon, R., Rice, M. M., Salisbury, M., John, C. (2011). A structured teamwork system to reduce clinical errors. In P. Spath (Ed.), *Error reduction in healthcare: A systems approach to improving patient safety* (2nd ed.). San Francisco: Jossey-Bass. (Chap. 14).

Slade, D., Scheeres, H., Manidis, M., Iedema, R., Dunston, R., Stein-Parbury, J., Matthiessen, C., Herke, M., McGregor, J. (2008). Emergency communication: The discursive challenges facing emergency clinicians and patients in hospital emergency departments. *Discourse & Communication, 2,* 271–298. doi:10.1177/1750481308091910.

Street, R. L. Jr., Makoul, G., Arora, N., & Epstein, R. M. (2009). How does communication heal? Pathways linking clinician-patient communication to health outcomes. *Patient Education and Counseling, 74,* 295–301.

Ternov, S. (n.d.). Learning for safety in health care and air traffic control. Lund University: PhD thesis.

Ternov, S. (2011). The human side of medicine mistakes. In P. Spath (Ed.), *Error reduction in healthcare: a systems approach to improving patient safety* (2nd ed.). San Francisco: Jossey-Bass. (Chap. 2)

US Government Accountability Office (GAO). (2004). *Veterans Affairs patient safety program: a cultural perspective of four medical facilities*. Washington: Report to the Secretary of Veterans Affairs.

Van Cott, H. (1994). Human errors: Their causes and reduction. In M. S. Bonger (Ed.), *Human error in medicine*. Hillsdale: Lawrence Erlbaum Associates.

World Health Organization (WHO) (2007). Conceptual framework for the international classification for patient safety Version 1.0 for use in field testing.

World Health Organization (WHO) (2013). The High 5s Project: Interim report. http://www.who.int/patientsafety/implementation/solutions/high5s/High5_InterimReport.pdf, Geneva, Switzerland. Accessed Sept 2014.

Chapter 5
Effective Clinician–Patient Communication: Strategies for Communicating Medical Knowledge

5.1 Introduction

Our work aimed to identify the communication strategies that the emergency department clinicians in our study used to manage individual patient journeys from triage to disposition, and to examine the impact of these spoken interactions on patient care. Emergency departments present many inherent challenges to communication because they are dynamic and noisy workplaces. Clinicians must make multiple decisions about many patients over very short time frames but are frequently interrupted and distracted in the process. Many patients who attend the emergency department are newcomers whose histories are not known to clinicians. Many present with atypical or vague symptoms, or with multiple comorbidities. Yet, both high demand and policy imperatives mean that clinicians are required to make decisions about diagnosis and treatment very quickly. Added to these difficulties, many emergency departments are used as training sites for junior doctors.

Our analysis of how clinicians and patients spoke, listened and responded to one another in emergency department interactions shows that two broad areas of communication affect the quality and safety of the patient journey through the emergency department:

- How medical knowledge and information is communicated
- How clinician–patient relationships are established and developed

It is our proposition that patient-centred care should reflect both these aspects. Overwhelmingly for the majority of clinicians we interviewed and observed, the priority was the transfer of medical knowledge and information; but both are essential components of effective communication and can occur simultaneously in every interaction. To deliver care effectively, clinicians must communicate care effectively.

In this chapter, we describe the strategies clinicians can use to effectively communicate medical knowledge. In the next chapter (Chap. 6), we summarise and

D. Slade et al., *Communicating in Hospital Emergency Departments,*
DOI 10.1007/978-3-662-46021-4_5

exemplify the strategies clinicians can use for establishing and developing a relationship with the patient, and by doing so involving them in their care. Both these essential aspects of effective communication occur simultaneously, but for the sake of description they are highlighted separately. In both chapters, we provide examples of each of the strategies, taken from the authentic extracts.

5.2   Bridging the Information Gap: Effective Strategies for Developing Shared Medical Knowledge and Decision-Making

In all stages of a patient's emergency department journey, clinicians must find out about the patient's medical condition and communicate medical information about this, and about the patient's management/treatment options. To do this effectively, clinicians need to be able to listen to the patient, impart medical information accurately and ensure the patient's awareness, understanding of and agreement to the treatment plan. The ability to listen to and validate the patient's experience is a key element of these strategies.

In this chapter, we outline eight strategies for developing shared medical knowledge and decision-making.

Table 5.1 gives examples of the eight communication strategies we identify:

1. Allowing space for the patient to tell their story
2. Seeking and recognising patient's knowledge and opinions about their condition
3. Explaining medical concepts clearly by moving between technical (medical) and common-sense (everyday) language
4. Spelling out explicitly the rationale for management/treatment options and decisions
5. Providing clear instructions for medication and other follow-up treatment, appointments
6. Explaining the hospital processes the patient will need to go through
7. Negotiating shared decision-making about treatment
8. Repeating key information, checking comprehension and offering clarification throughout

Below we discuss each strategy in detail.

5.2.1   Make Space for the Patient's Story

Many clinicians are aware that it is an effective diagnostic strategy to give the patient the space to tell the story of their illness and injury. After all, patients are the most valuable source of information about themselves. However, less confident (often more junior) clinicians can sometimes deny the patient this valuable com-

Table 5.1 Strategies for developing shared medical knowledge and decision-making

Communication strategy	Description	Examples from authentic recorded interactions
Make space for the patient to tell their story	Initially open up the space for patients to talk by asking open, neutral questions	'Now what seems to be the problem?' 'And how can I help you today?'
Seek and recognise the patient's knowledge and opinions about their condition	Facilitate the knowledge building process by eliciting and valuing patients' knowledge about their case and prior treatments	'So it was yesterday afternoon you were passing these big clots. Were they red, or did they look black like that?'
	Normalise patients' medical symptoms and concerns about what is happening to them	'There's a few things that can cause bleeding out the bum. I think in you the most likely thing is that it's coming from some diverticular disease. And sometimes little pockets on the wall of the bowel can bleed from time to time and they can get infected'
Explain medical concepts clearly by moving between technical (medical) and common-sense (everyday) language	Limit technical language or jargon and explain terms that patients might not understand	'What we have there is what we call epididymo-orchitis. That's just our fancy way of saying infection'
Spell out explicitly the rationale for management/treatment options and decisions	Provide patients with clear reasons for ongoing treatment or management plans	'Now, we need to rule out a problem with the aorta, which is the big blood vessel coming in the top of your heart. And the only way to do that is to do a CT scan'
	Wherever appropriate, make the reasoning process available to patients	'Hopefully we won't have to do the X-ray again. But we may have to because the situation changes on different days'
	Explain the sequence and priority of treatments	'Alright, but for now the priority is treating the infection. Make sure there is nothing nasty with the biopsy and then we can talk about how to get the waterworks better in the long term'
Provide clear instructions for medication and other follow-up treatment, appointments, etc.	State instructions clearly and repeat or ask patients to repeat to confirm comprehension	'I wouldn't use anti-inflammatory tablets at the moment because they could make you bleed from the prostate, so take Panadol—two tablets every 4 hrs. So that's a maximum of eight tablets per day. OK?'
Signpost the hospital processes the patient will need to go through	Set out the steps the patient is likely to go through and the different demands that will be made of him/her	'I'll send you up to the next window just to give your Medicare details and things. And then one of our doctors is going to call you through the house doctor section today, so they'll bring you through and have a chat to you…'

Table 5.1 (continued)

Communication strategy	Description	Examples from authentic recorded interactions
Negotiate shared decision-making about treatment	Encourage patients to debate, clarify and discuss their treatment options	'If the bandage falls off you might want to try something simpler? So we could try the one you used last time, if you like'
	Encourage patients to comply with recommended treatment plans by negotiating preferred treatment plans with them	'If the bleeding continues then we'll consider doing something else. OK? So what are our options? Well, the definitive option is radiotherapy'
Repeat key information, check comprehension and offer clarification throughout	Continually check that patients have understood and offer the opportunity for them to ask for clarification. Confirm comprehension and agreement with recommended treatment plans	'When you fell down onto that bone, the coccyx bone it's a very thin area and it's going to be sore. The bruising is going to be…the pain itself will probable last for at least a week. It's going to be very, very sore'

municative opportunity. While we acknowledge that clinicians are under pressure to set the agenda in the emergency department, our data indicate that allowing patients a greater opportunity to contribute to building shared knowledge may be a way of making the patient journey more efficient, because patients more often than not provide crucial medical information themselves. At the same time, patients have the satisfaction of knowing that they have been given the opportunity to discuss their concerns and anxieties and explain what they think may be wrong with them.

Indicators of whether the patient has been given sufficient space to tell their story are the use of particular types of questions, the type and number of initiating utterances made by the patient, the type and number of clarifications and queries, both by the patient and the clinician, and the length of patient turns during talking. An additional indication is to what degree the clinician expands on and enhances the information the patient provides and picks up on the patient cues.

Here is an example of a triage nurse starting her assessment by asking the patient an open question ('Um, so what's happened today?). She then gives the patient the space to provide a detailed narrative, using minimal acknowledgements (such as 'yeah' and 'mm') and asks more specific questions when she needs further clarification:

Nurse: Yeah. Yeah. Um, so what's happened today?
Patient: Um, I'm unwell sort of like as he said for days but this is different.
Nurse: Why is he giving you penicillin, just for an upper respiratory tract infection or something is it?
Patient: I don't know. I've been—had like a virus and tonsillitis and then pharyngitis.

Nurse: Tonsillitis. OK.

Patient: And then, um, had to go to my after hours 'cause I couldn't get into my doctor's. And after hours doctor gave me that one.

Nurse: Yeah.

Patient: So I started taking that by itself. I have had an allergic reaction to Keflex before.

Nurse: Mm.

Patient: But this isn't Keflex. So I—I had it and there was no allergic reaction to that. Was on it for a couple of days and wasn't getting better. Went to my doctor and he had one look at me and said 'Shit, you don't look well'. I was not well, I couldn't—have not moved for four days or ate or drink.

Nurse: Mm.

Patient: And he said bend over, and gave me a shot in my bum, gave me—said they're not strong enough, gave me a shot straight in the bum.

Nurse: Mm.

Patient: So last night I sweated all night, all night sweating. I thought oh, I'm finally going to break it, thank God. And this morning I went—I've had a temperature for five days, non-stop—um, ( ) this morning I felt a tiny bit better.

Nurse: Mm.

———

Patient: My face was going cold and numb

Nurse: Mm.

Patient: Felt like it was cold, um, like ice cold water running down from my neck, or down ( ) it sounds very ( ) but that's the only way I can explain it.

Nurse: Yeah.

Patient: It's the only way I can explain it, like cold, numb, just seeing little black dots and stuff.

Nurse: Mm.

Patient: And was this white frothy stuff was coming out, bits of white froth.

Nurse: Yeah.

Patient: And um, when I had a allergic reaction to Keflex, I had the white frothy thing too. So…

Nurse: OK.

Patient: I thought I'd just wear it out for a while. So I was laying in bed and thinking I'll get better, it'll go, it'll go…

In the next extract, the doctor gives the patient space to provide the information he needs. He offers the patient space to provide an alternative in his first question and then uses assumptive questions to show he is listening and to probe for further clarification:

Doctor: Um and at home do you need any oxygen? Or…

Patient: No, um, ( ) Ventolin inhaler thing.

Doctor: OK.

Patient: Ah, I was on Symbicort there, ah, Spiriva, is that another ( )?

Doctor: It is.

Patient: But the Ventolin he seems to have put me on and then uh, um the steroids.

Doctor: OK.

Patient: And, ah, the Vibramycin is the one, I'd say that has released all this mucous ==

Doctor: == And so you are coughing up—you are coughing up gunk? [assumptive question]

Patient: Oh, I have got yellow.

Doctor: Yellow.

Patient: When it comes up. There seems to be a hell of a lot here that's not == coming.

Doctor: == So you feel like—you feel like it's there? [assumptive question]

Patient: I feel like it's there.

Doctor: But you can't get all of it up? [assumptive question]

Patient: I can't.

Doctor: OK.

Patient: I've never been one to really be able to cough == up.

In contrast, in the excerpt below, the nurse begins with two open questions, but then does not allow space for the patient to tell his story, as many of the questions she asks are closed (requiring a yes/no answer):

Patient: == Some might say it would be easier.

N3: Yeah, so how far are you affected, in bowels and bladder or? [open question]

Patient: Ah, well…

N3: Not quite, or ( ). How long have you had [ ] for?

Patient: Ah, since '91.

N3: (Was it) a kind of rapid onset for you? [closed question]

Patient: Oh, no, gradual.

N3: Oh, ( ) alright ( ).

N3: What specialist looks after you?

Patient: Oh, B.

N3: OK, yeah. You're not on steroids at the moment? [closed question]

Patient: No.

N3: Not allergic to anything? [closed question]

Patient: Ah, yeah.

N3: Oh, OK.

Patient: Pred—Prednisolone.

N3: Oh, are you? [closed question]

Patient: And Keflex.

N3: ( ) what they treat you all the time with? OK, now do I need to == ( )? [closed question]

Patient: == Yes, please.

N3: OK.

N3: I wish I could help you more (but).

Table 5.2 Contrasting more and less effective ways to elicit the patient's story

More effective (Jean)	Less effective (Graydon)
Nurse: And you're here today for…? [open question]	*Nurse: Were you in here yesterday were you? [closed question]*
Patient: I um had some stitches put in on Sunday and it was sort of a tricky little uh cut, so they wanted me to come back today just to check on it.	*Patient: Yes, very early yesterday morning.*
Nurse: OK. And how's the pain been in the leg?	*Nurse: And what was the problem then? [open question]*
Patient: It's OK. You know…you know it's there but it's not throbbing or anything.	*Patient: Um…oh well…*
Nurse: Not too bad? OK. And you haven't noticed any redness or anything around the area?	*Relative: Same problem*
Patient: Well I haven't taken it off.	*Patient: Same problem, but um…*
	Nurse: Yeah, it's just that I'm different so I'm asking the same sort of questions ==
	Patient: Oh right.
	Nurse: So I can triage you, that's all.
	Patient: That's alright. Um…so yeah, we went through um…blood tests, ECG, um…X-ray. They couldn't ah…the doctors at the time, they couldn't see anything acute…. And he said er…there's a problem. Mmm…. Basically what he's saying was that er…. Is it the…is it the left ventricle?
	Relative: It's ah…yeah…he's ah…he's in heart failure basically.
	Nurse: Mmhm. How old are you?
	Patient: Fifty-one.
	Nurse: Allergic to anything?
	Patient: No.
	Nurse: You on medication…at the moment?
In this example, the triage nurse opened up the space for the patient to tell her what she knew about her injury by asking an open question. The focus of the questions narrowed as the nurse checked her understanding of Jean's (review suture for leg injury) level of pain ('Not too bad'). She then used an assumptive question ('And you haven't noticed any redness or anything around the area?') to check for evidence of infection. The continued use of 'and' at the beginning of each question created a sense of continuity in the questioning process.	*In this example, the triage nurse opened with a closed question followed by an open question. The triage nurse initially established that Graydon (cardiology admission) had presented at the emergency department the day before. When she asked what the problem had been then (i.e. the day before), Graydon and his wife assumed that this information would be on record. Graydon and his wife were unaware that the same process is initiated for each patient who presents at the emergency department, even if they have attended the emergency department as recently as the day before.*

Table 5.2 gives examples from triage conversations with Jean (review suture for leg injury) and Graydon (cardiology admission) and discusses why we believe one interaction is more effective than the other.

In Graydon's case, the nurse asked only five questions during triage. Four of these related to the patient's medical condition and one to the hospital system. Graydon asked only one question about his medical condition. His main contribution to the interview was to respond to the questions he was asked. Although one of

Graydon's responses as well as one of his wife's were more lengthy because they had been through the same process the day before and they were now more familiar with the system, they were constrained in terms of the space they were allowed. Having been told that Graydon was in heart failure, the triage nurse responded with 'Mmhm' and proceeded to ask another two questions about his age and allergies.

The triage nurse explained the reason she needed to reassess the presenting illness herself, and the patient and his wife responded by sharing what they knew. Once the presenting condition was established, the triage nurse returned to the triage protocol, even though this information would have been recorded in the patient's notes. This is a demonstration of the fact that all clinicians are accountable for their own practice and must stick to protocols—but it is frequently mystifying to patients who assume clinicians have access to prior information.

At the conclusion of the triage interview, the triage nurse told the patient that he was to be placed in the acute section of the emergency department, and then took him to the bed and began the admission stage herself. She then double-checked the patient's personal details, and reaffirmed her own responsibility for this when the patient appeared bemused:

N: And you said you're not allergic to anything?
Patient: No.
Nurse: And your date of birth is [date of birth removed]?
Patient: That's correct. [sound of crashing] Should've left the...tag on from yesterday, shouldn't I?
Relative: Yeah.
Nurse: It wouldn't count.

Some doctors in our consultations opened space for patients to tell their stories very effectively in the initial medical consultation stage. In the example below, the doctor gives space to Jean to outline her condition.

Doctor: So, what seems to be the problem now?
Patient: Well nothing's the problem. I came in on Sunday.
Doctor: Mm hm.
Patient: I had a very deep cut in my leg ==
Doctor: Mm hm.
Patient: == and I came in the ambulance because it was bleeding a lot ==
Doctor: Mm hm.
Patient: == and ah, then [name removed], or the doctor, ==
Doctor: Mm hm.
Patient: == She.... It was har...difficult to sort of stitch because of the ==
Doctor: Mm hm.
Patient: == because of the shape of it and everything ==
Doctor: Mm hm.
Patient: == So, um, she just wanted me to come and have the dressing changed today and to check that everything was going OK.
Doctor: Mm, OK, good.

In this example, the doctor initially engaged the patient by asking an open, neutral question. She then limited her own contributions so that Jean could describe the sequence of events uninterrupted. The doctor's response at the end of the narrative was positive but non-committal, 'Mm, OK, good'.

In Chap. 4, we quoted from the case of Fahime (dizziness, feeling stressed), the Middle Eastern patient who was examined by two junior doctors, neither of whom picked up on clues to her depression. In fact, in the 3 hrs Fahime spent in the emergency department, she was asked 149 questions, most of which were closed (requiring only yes/no answers). By contrast, Fahime and her family asked a total of four questions, suggesting a striking lack of collaboration in the patient–clinician relationship.

Our data repeatedly indicate that allowing patients a greater opportunity to contribute to shared-knowledge building may be a way of making the patient journey more efficient. Patients may well be able to provide crucial medical information. This is particularly the case in the initial medical consultation stage. If clinicians allow patients room to tell their stories, by encouraging longer turns at talking, patients may provide crucial medical information themselves. At the same time, patients have the satisfaction of knowing that they have been given the opportunity to express themselves. However, given the time and clinical pressures on senior doctors, they must find out efficiently what they need to know from patients.

Some doctors—mainly senior doctors—displayed considerable skill in allowing the patient time to talk while also narrowing in to clarify essential medical information. For example, the two senior doctors involved in the diagnosis stage for Nola (per-rectal (PR) bleeding) and Graydon (cardiology admission) used the same strategy that other clinicians in our data have employed, and began the final history-taking process by asking an open, neutral question, i.e. 'What were you doing at the time?' (Nola); 'Can you tell me what it was like?' (Graydon) This offers the patient communication space. They then made use of a range of question types based on the information they needed to establish a plausible diagnosis/hypothesis.

The surgical registrar who took responsibility for care of Nola during the diagnosis, treatment and disposition stage of her consultation invited Nola to tell her story:

D3: What were you doing at the time?
Patient: Well nothing really. I—I'd just had lunch and I was, um, I'd had this green apple, oh well Granny Smith apple, and ah, I thought oh, that was giving me the pains in me tummy. Anyway, ah, so I thought oh, I better go to the loo.

The doctor checked that some of the information Nola had given in the initial medical consultation was still the case, by asking a series of assumptive questions. This less direct style of questioning appeared to place a positive value on Nola's earlier contribution. The re-questioning process gave Nola an opportunity to explain the reason why she did not have a scheduled colonoscopy, and time to accept the inevitable need for another one in the future:

D3: So you had some, ah, some tummy pains first?
Patient: Just—just slight, you know, and I thought oh that's that green apple. When I got there, though, mm, it come away and then I felt faint and called to my husband.

D3: So you felt like you had to go in a hurry?

Patient: No, not really. It was, um, just that I was just gonna go anyway…

———

D3: You mention that you felt faint as well?

Patient: Oh, yes. Yes, I felt as if I was gonna faint. That's when I called out to my husband because if I fell I'd hit my head on the hand basin and all that 'cause it's all so close, you know.

D3: OK.

Patient: So, anyway, anyway…

———

D3: You had some diarrhoea, some bloating and some pain?

Patient: Mm. Is that what that says there is it? [patient notes]

D3: Dr ( ). [muttering while reading notes]

Patient: No, but as soon as I ( ) blood came I thought, this is it, I need another colonoscopy. But I hate that lead up to it, you know, that's why I sort of put it off from having another one.

D3: You were supposed to have another one and you never did. And it was nine years ago now?

Patient: Nine years is it?

D3: Nine years.

Patient: From whom?

D3: That was when you had the colonoscopy, was in 1999?

When the surgical registrar required more specific information, he asked a series of closed questions, often repeating what Nola said out loud, gradually building up a clearer picture of the problem for himself and for her:

D3: And did you actually pass, ah… [closed question]

Patient: Oh, yes. Yes. Clots, about that big, mm.

D3: Ah-hm.

Patient: Dark.

D3: Can you—yeah, describe them to me? They were dark? [closed question]

Patient: Dark.

D3: Big clots? [closed question]

Patient: Clots of blood, mm.

D3: OK.

Patient: How can you describe that?

D3: Oh well, just the colour, the size, I suppose.

Patient: Yeah, clots. (Attempt to get more information from P)

D3: Did you do poo with it as well? [closed question]

Patient: Ah, no. That—that was all that came.

D3: It was just blood? [closed question]

Patient: Yes. A lot of it too.

D3: Oh, OK. Alright.

In Graydon's case (cardiology admission), the senior staff specialist used a series of very specific, largely closed questions to focus on particular aspects of Graydon's history. Graydon's case was potentially very serious, so there was a sense of urgency in the interaction that precluded any negotiation around treatment. In the following examples, the doctor is focused on the patient's pain. Her questions follow the classic two or three-turn pattern described by Mishler (1984) in which the doctor asks a question, the patient responds, and then usually the doctor briefly acknowledges the response before asking the next question and so on. In other words, the doctor has complete control of the interaction:

Doctor: Can you tell me...what was it like? Can you describe it at all?
Patient: I've tried this before...um.... Not really sharp but...acute.
Doctor: OK.
Patient: Um...and...consistent?
Doctor: Did it go anywhere else other than across your back?
Patient: No.
Doctor: OK. [three-turn pattern] And was it absolutely non-stop? Or did it come in waves?
Patient: No, it was non-stop.
Doctor: OK. [three-turn pattern]And how did it get better? Did it gradually get better?
Patient: Yeah. It um...seemed to dissipate from the outside and took...at one stage, ()...
Doctor: OK. [three-turn pattern] And then did it go away...completely?
Patient: Yeah. [two-turn pattern]
Doctor: How long did it last...about?
Patient: I'd say altogether somewhere between two and a half to three hours.
Doctor: Oh [three-turn pattern]. And have you ever had a pain like that before?
Patient: No. [two-turn pattern]

Graydon's main contribution was through the information he provided about his medical history: his answers (89) to which his wife added 15 and his 63 statements (43 about his illness and 20 about the system). Graydon's wife added information to the shared knowledge by contributing 15 answers about Graydon's medical history and 24 statements (11 about his illness and 13 about the system). Most of the questions asked, by both the doctor (59 out of 91) and the nurse (6 out of 6), were closed questions, which limited the scope of Graydon's answers to a 'yes' or a 'no'.

5.2.2 Recognise the Patient's Knowledge and Opinions About Their Condition

Giving the patient space includes not just asking for but also respecting the patient's opinion of his or her condition. The most effective clinicians listen actively to their patients' accounts and validate the patient's contribution to the consultation. Here is one doctor doing this with another patient:

Doctor: OK. Um, have you felt like you've had fevers?

Patient: Ah, that day I had, and I've been taking Panadol and stuff for that…. I'm alright now.

Doctor: Do you think the Clindamycin has made a difference == to the rest of you but…?

Patient: == Yeah. I think it's done…yeah, done well for my leg and it's just

Doctor: OK.

Patient: Panadol and stuff, just kind've done alright.

———-

Patient: == Ah, sometimes I have headaches, um…

Doctor: Associated with this…this episode do you think?

Patient: Yeah, I have in the—the last nine days.

Doctor: OK.

When a clinician does allow the patient space to tell her story, the clinician can then intervene in the narrative at relevant points to clarify what the patient already knows about her condition. Failure to hear the story tends to lead to failure to find out useful information the patient could share, if encouraged to.

In the following examples, although both nurses use assumptive and closed questions, in the more effective example, nurse 2 (N2) alternatively allows space to Nola (PR bleeding), and occasionally homes in on a detail. On the other hand, N2 in the less effective example continues with closed and multiple questions and then follows these with questions, all of which limit Chaitali (PV bleeding) in giving a proper account of her illness (Table 5.3).

Simply finding out what the patient knows is useful. However, it is even more effective for the clinician to actively demonstrate empathy and understanding, thereby validating the patient's collaborative contribution to the consultation.

In the extracts below, we see the junior doctor with Donna (HX, anal fissure), seeking information about her condition and what she has experienced. The junior doctor valued Donna's input into the discussion by first allowing Donna to add further information about the time frame and development of the haemorrhoids. She asked additional questions about Donna's symptoms and experiences, listening attentively ('Yes, Yeah, OK, OK. Mm') and valuing her understanding of what the patient experienced. As the patient was in considerable pain, she also expressed her sympathy ('I'm feeling for you'):

Doctor: OK so tell me when this problem first started Donna.

Patient: I'd say it's probably about a month, probably about—I had a haemorrhoid.

Doctor: Yeah.

Patient: And I had that lanced a couple of weeks ago.

Doctor: Yeah.

Patient: == And, um—

Doctor: I'm feeling == for you.

Patient: == but I thought that it was more than just a haemorrhoid.

Doctor: Yeah.

Patient: And when that cleared up then ==

Table 5.3 Contrasting more and less effective ways to recognise the patient's knowledge

More effective (Nola)	Less effective (Chaitali)
Nurse: So you've been leak—bleeding a lot have you? [Assumptive question] *Patient: Well I consider it's a lot.* *Nurse: Is it in the stool or around the stool when you open your bowels? [Closed question]* *Patient: Um…I haven't had a bowel movement. It all started yesterday.* *Nurse: Yep. [Allows space to continue]* *Patient: I had an apple, a Granny Smith apple, and I thought oh, the pains, I thought it's that sour Granny Smith.* *Nurse: [Laughs]* *Patient: Anyway, I went to the loo…* *Nurse: Yep. [Allows space to continue]* *Patient: And I could feel myself, coming out in a real sweat and I called to my husband 'cause I thought I was going to faint and fall against the, you know, the basin and that.* *Nurse: Yes, yep. [Allows space to continue]* *Patient: And—and then—and I'm perspiring, something terrible ==* *Nurse: == Mm mm [Allows space to continue]* *Patient: == really big clots like that.* *Nurse: Yeah, so big clots. [Allows space to continue]* *Patient: Yes, they were.* *Nurse: OK. Have you been constipated? [Closed question]* *Patient: No not today.* *Nurse: Have you been constipated? Just lie yourself back.* *Patient: Oh my bowels have never been really good I don't think.* *Nurse: Oh OK. [Allows space to continue]* *Patient: Ever.* *Nurse: And have you had this before, in the past? [Closed question]* *Patient: Not with the bleeding.* *Nurse: No? OK. Alright*	*Nurse: So now you've come in with bleeding since this morning? [Assumptive question]* *Patient: I—I was here actually last week. [Voice distant from mic]* *Nurse: Yeah, what time did you—did you just wake up and you were already bleeding? When you went to bed last night you were OK? [Assumptive question and multiple questions]* *Patient: No, I also have the bleeding, but ( ) never ( ).* *Nurse: Since your treatment, yeah? [Assumptive question]* *Patient: Yeah, but this morning there were clots.* *Nurse: You're passing clots into a pad? [Assumptive question]. Have you got any pain at the moment? [Multiple questions]* *Patient: Little bit.* *Nurse: What would you say it was out of 10 ( )?* *Patient: Pardon?* *Nurse: What would the pain be out of 10? Ten being hit by a truck, and zero, no pain. What would you say?* *Patient: About eight.* *Nurse: Eight. Have you had anything before you came in for pain at all? [Closed question]* *……………* *Nurse: ( ). Are you allergic to anything at the moment? [Closed question]* *Patient: Just codeine.* *Nurse: Codeine?* *Patient: Yeah.* *Nurse: OK. And apart from your obviously, um, ovarian cancer, have you got any heart or lung problems? [Closed and double question]* *Patient: No, I'm asthmatic,* *Nurse: Asthmatic* *Patient: And osteoporosis, osteoporosis in my neck, pain in my neck [Chuckles]*

Table 5.3 (continued)

More effective (Nola)	Less effective (Chaitali)
In this example, nurse 2 briefly reviewed her understanding of why Nola (PR bleeding) had presented to the emergency department. She first checked why Nola had come to the emergency department by asking her an assumptive question ('So you've been leak— bleeding a lot have you'), and then allowed her the space to provide a detailed narrative during longer turns of talk. The nurse responded to Nola's story with minimal acknowledgements (such as 'Yep' and 'Mm mm') as a way of encouraging her to tell all she knew, and asked more specific questions when she needed further clarification. Nurse 2 kept the patient's direct experience in focus, by using the personal pronoun 'you'. Nola in turn, responded by giving a very personal and detailed account of what had happened, from the perspective of 'I'	*In this example, an agency nurse settling Chaitali (PV bleeding) used several closed questions, assumptive questions and multiple questions all of which restricted space for Chaitali to respond. The question on the severity of pain is a standard one, but was initially misunderstood by Chaitali whose first language was not English. As Chaitali was in extreme pain, we would argue that the reference to the truck was also extremely inappropriate, as was the way in which nurse 2 referred to her 'obviously, um, ovarian cancer'*

Doctor: == Yeah.

Patient: —yeah this fissure's just gradually got worse.

Doctor: Yeah, OK. So how long ago did the haemorrhoid sort of develop?

Patient: I think only five weeks ago.

Doctor: OK, and had you had haemorrhoids in the past or was this a new thing for you?

Patient: Yeah look I've had a haemorrhoid when I had my kids.

Doctor: Yeah, OK.

Patient: So that's 19 years ago.

Doctor: Yeah.

Patient: Yeah no, it's—but a fissure, I was in here, um, September 2007.

Doctor: Yeah.

Patient: With a fissure for five days.

Doctor: OK. And the um—do you know whether it was an internal one or an external one?

Patient: Oh it's just—just sort of in—it's just inside.

Doctor: OK. And was it ==

Patient: == So it's that spot.

5.2.3   Explain Medical Concepts in Common-sense Language

One of the challenges clinicians face is that they must diagnose using scientific understandings and terminology but communicate with patients who do not 'speak' the biomedical discourse. Effective clinician communicators learn to translate complex medical concepts and terminology into vernacular language that patients can understand. Clinicians can help patients register and retain information—firstly, by considering what information is important from the patient's point of view; secondly, by ensuring they use everyday terminology where appropriate; and thirdly, by repeating key facts at different times.

In the following example, the senior registrar communicated his medical knowledge and his diagnosis to patient Nola (PR bleeding) by describing her condition in terms that she could understand. He also explained the medical consequences of her condition, and thus provided a clear rationale for his treatment plan:

D3: There's a few things that can cause bleeding out the bum. I think in you the most likely is that it's coming from some diverticular disease. Now that means little pockets on the wall of the bowel that they've noticed before when they've done your colonoscopies.
Patient: Have they?
D3: Yeah. It's not a serious problem, it's not like cancer. But these little pockets on the wall of the bowel can bleed from time to time and they can get infected.
Patient: Oh.
D3: And I suspect that yours are bleeding. So we need to—there's no um specific surgery that we need to do, but we do need to bring you in to hospital to keep an eye on you until the bleeding settles down. And then once it's all settled down we, um, will do...plan another colonoscopy.

We see the same skill demonstrated by the senior doctor responsible for Graydon (cardiology admission):

Doctor: Just because it's...when it doesn't work well, it sort of backs up into your lungs. So you need to stay in hospital, OK? We're going to put you on some water pill, which is going to make you pee like a racehorse.

In some cases, clinicians provide the correct medical terminology as well as using an everyday gloss of a patient's condition. For example:

Patient: I've worked out 15 operations since I was five, and that was tonsillitis the first.
Nurse: So you've had a tonsillectomy? The tonsils out?

5.2.4   Spell Out Explicitly Management/Treatment Rationales

An important role of emergency department clinicians is to provide patients with clear information about their medical conditions and their ongoing testing, treatment and management plans. Some clinicians make their reasoning processes available to the patient. By including patients in this way, clinicians can provide patients with crucial knowledge, which gives them the opportunity to participate in making decisions.

In the following example, the doctor explains to the patient what he could see on her X-ray and why he was thinking of taking various options:

Doctor: Well, ma'am, OK. Madam, I'm just going to explain to you. You can see the fracture clearly == here.

Patient: == Yes, I totally can.

Doctor: It—it looks like in a good position from there. I'm going to talk to one of the senior doctors here just to get her opinion. But usually for such kind of fractures, what we do, we put a half cast.

Patient: Yes, this is what my GP thought it would be.

Doctor: Ah, let me have a look at the other leg. Sorry, madam, just to compare. Yeah, this one is a bit swollen. I believe the swelling is related to the fracture.

Patient: Yes.

Doctor: OK.

Patient: Yes.

Doctor: So actually a full cast at the moment...

Patient: Yes.

Doctor: ...within a few days this swelling is going to be subsided,: == getting down.

Patient: == Yes, it will, yes.

Doctor: And the full cast it going to be really loose.

Patient: And that won't be == any use.

Doctor: == And it's going to be—it's going to be useless.

Patient: Exactly.

Doctor: So what we do is a half cast, get this swelling subsided.

Patient: Yes.

Doctor: And then give it seven days and then I'm going to give you a referral to the fracture clinic.

Patient: Right.

Doctor: You will need to ring, get an appointment done and come [P Yes]—come the day of the appointment you will be seen by the specialist people, ortho wards, and they—they will get a full cast done and give you the good advice.

As already mentioned, explaining medical knowledge clearly typically involves moving between technical and everyday terminology, as the nurse in the following example demonstrates. She also explains the medical consequences of the patient's condition and thus provides a clear rationale for his treatment plan:

Patient: Dr C did explain sort of briefly, um, the other day, like it's a sort of form of herpes. But sort of, no, not really?

Nurse: Yeah, well...

Patient: With a different sort of...

Nurse: Yeah.

Patient: ...strain.

Nurse: Chicken pox.

Patient: Chicken pox.

Nurse: It's called Varicella zoster.

Patient: Oh, OK.

Nurse: Herpes Varicella zoster so we just call it HVZ, but it's not…
Patient: HVZ.
Nurse: It's chicken pox.
Patient: It's chicken pox.
Nurse: And the—and the silly name for it is that. But, we always go with the friendliest name, not the most unfriendliest name.
Patient: [Chuckles]
Nurse: We go. So it's a virus.
Patient: Mm-hm.
Nurse: It's part of the herpes virus family, called shingles.
Patient: Oh, OK.
Nurse: Ah, three trigeminal ganglions which is pretty much your arm, == and chest…
Patient: == Oh, OK, arm and chest.
Nurse: …and your back.
Patient: Right.
Nurse: So it follows that nerve route.
Patient: Oh, OK.
Nurse: So it's a typical picture.
Patient: Yeah.
Nurse: Ah, features. Has a rash. Painful, lasts 10–15 days. [P Mm mm] You have a kind of cold or a—feel as though you've got a cold for 48–72 hrs before it…

In the following example, the triage nurse explains her reasoning about the patient's high blood pressure very clearly to her:

Nurse: Swap arms and we'll just measure this one. OK. Keep that nice and straight like so. So that one is 218, that reading. Um So it is up a little bit. Years ago we used to have a little capsule and it had a medication in it. We'd put a hole in it, squirt it under your tongue and it'd drop your blood pressure very, very quickly. Ah, that was about 15 years ago because we were very concerned == your blood pressure is up…
Patient: == Ah, yeah.
Nurse: …would you pop a blood vessel in == your head and have a stroke?
Patient: == Yeah, yes. Yeah, that's why we don't…
Nurse: Or, would it cause lots of problems elsewhere in your body? We don't–the evidence now shows that blood pressure should be very, very carefully dropped. And that tends to be not over a 24 hrs period even, it can be for longer. So we very rarely will, even with the blood pressure of 236, we'll have patients with blood pressures higher than that, and we will actually look at starting you on some kind of blood pressure tablets with your GP following it up because we only get to see you once usually. That's good for you.

Some clinicians explain their reasoning to the patient. This allows clinicians to provide patients with crucial knowledge, which gives them the opportunity to contribute to decision-making.

In the next extract from the consultation with Jack (multiple sclerosis, feeling unwell, weak), the senior doctor explained very clearly to Jack his reasoning, what he was thinking and why he was choosing. Although he could not assist Jack further medically, he recognised that Jack required additional assistance:

Doctor: Yeah. OK. Well, listen, I guess in terms of the results that we see, they look fine, OK. Your blood count is completely normal, inflammatory markers are not exciting. There's nothing that would suggest that you've got an underlying infection or anything, which is always a worry with the symptoms that you're describing.

Patient: It is for me, yeah.

Doctor: Um, and you know, everything from that point of view looks alright. My bigger concern probably is that, you know, you've got a disease that is scary and all the things that you're describing are probably, you know, kind of mentally consistent with you being under quite a bit of stress with all of this. Um...

Patient: Yeah.

Doctor: Which I think may be part of this. Um.

Patient: Yeah.

Doctor: And you know, I guess in terms of following that up, perhaps [your specialist] and his bread and butter world, you know, you've got [ ], these are the symptoms of [ ], you carry on.

Patient: Yeah, yeah.

Doctor: Um, but the question is whether there may be more help in terms of getting, you know, one of our psychologists or social workers,

Patient: Yeah.

Doctor: Somebody to put you in contact with the network, you know, 'cause it sounds like you want answers and...

In the following example, the senior doctor admits that she cannot explain the patient's pain at that moment, but she shows herself willing to give her medical opinion, based on her extensive medical experience. At the same time, she provides a clear rationale for why the patient needs to stay in hospital:

Doctor: I think though...I can't explain this pain that you had in your back, so my gut feeling is...that it was muscular from the coughing thing. I...I think that's probably what it was...because usually when you have a split in your big blood vessel in your chest...very bad things happen...and...maybe it went away and you're the same as you always were. But I can't say for sure that's not the case.

Patient: Mmhm,

Doctor: The other thing is that your heart muscle is not working very well and that's why your breathing is bad.

Patient: Yeah.

Doctor: Just because it's...when it doesn't work well, it sort of backs up into your lungs. So you need to stay in hospital, OK?

Explaining clearly is essential when a patient is being asked to consent to extensive tests. The following two extracts from the consultation with Graydon (cardiology admission), show the lengths to which the doctor needed to go in order to provide the patient with sufficient information before the patient could agree to have the tests. However, the 'payback' for the communicative effort was that Graydon indicated not only that he was willing to have the tests but also that he understood that they were important:

Doctor: We may also want to do some more imaging…studies here. Not right here…
*   back in the radiology department, but er—( ) cardiologist.*
Patient: OK.
Doctor: But I'll get ( ) cardiologist one, and ( ) make a plan between us as to where
*   this is going and when…and what makes sense. Is that alright?*
Patient: Sounds great. Yeah.

———

Doctor: But um…I'll go and go through all this and as soon as I know what's going
*   to happen with the cardiology and with the next lot of tests, I'll come back and*
*   give you a shout.*
Patient: Alright.
Doctor: I'll speak to you soon Sir…

———

Doctor: I just talked to my boss and she agrees with me that we need to do some
*   rather more extensive imaging on top of your chest X-ray. What we'd like to do*
*   is a CT scan of your chest and abdomen because we'd like to look at particularly*
*   the condition of your aorta which is the big blood vessel coming in the top of*
*   the heart. Runs up to the heart, all the way down the side of your chest and your*
*   abdomen and down to your legs.*
Patient: OK.
Doctor: Now, we need to rule out a problem with the aorta as the cause of the pain
*   down in your belly and your groin. And the only way to do that is to do a CT scan*
*   with and without the contrast injection. Now, contrast injections sometimes can*
*   cause a reaction. It's unusual. Have you ever had a CT scan before?*
Patient: Never.

———

Doctor: I think on the—in the balance of risk and benefit in the situation is over-
*   whelming on the side of…*
Patient: The CT scan's going to be, ah, important.
Doctor: Yes. I think it's an important thing to do. Um…
Patient: Alright.

5.2.5   Provide Clear Instructions for Medication and Other Follow-Up Treatment

Part of providing patient-centred care in the emergency department involves making sure the patient has clear instructions about medication and other follow-up treatment or appointments. This has a direct relationship to patient safety as discussed in Chap. 1 (see, for example, Buckley et al. 2013).

In the following example, the doctor provides clear instructions for the management and follow-up treatment of the patient's wound:

Doctor: And hopefully tomorrow it shouldn't happen because you're off (the rest of the) stuff, going—morphines are off your system, [medication] is off your system and it's Endone only, so it's not too much.
Patient: OK, yeah. What's in that? Is that morphine?
Doctor: It's morphine-like.
Patient: Yeah.
Doctor: But orally active.
Patient: Yeah.
Doctor: It acts for four hours at a time, so it's pretty good. So your regimen will be Panadol four times a day.
Patient: Yeah.
Doctor: Your Voltaren, two to three times a day with food.
Patient: Yes.
Doctor: There's Endone, I would think since you are in pain, four times.
Patient: Right.
Doctor: But you wanna cut that back, you're fine, you're sleeping, so don't wake up for that, you can miss it.
Patient: Yep.
Doctor: And Mon—Tues—Thursday, go to her, and then see how you are going then. She's otherwise also a good person to go to GP to start off with. I've told her your problem…
Patient: Yup, OK.
Doctor: …so you need to have some referrals to take to her.
Patient: Yeah, OK.
Doctor: OK?
Patient: Alright, thank you.

When the patient's first language is not English, effective clinicians take extra care to ensure their instructions have been understood, as we see in this example with Luca (stiff neck), whose first language was not English:

N: So once that's done, you should probably use some pain relief or…
Patient: Um
N: You've got some at home?
Patient: I've got Nurofen Plus so.
N: Oh, OK. Just make sure you um, have that with some food, yeah.

The doctor then goes on to say:

Doctor: I wouldn't be using anti-inflammatory tablets at the moment because they could make you bleed from the…prostate =
Patient: = Yes, yes, yes. But I used Panamax. Four tablets = last week.

Doctor: = Yeah. You must…. No, yeah. But that's not enough.
Patient: That's not enough!
Doctor: You need to take two…every four hours.
Patient: Ohhh!
Doctor: A maximum of eight per day.
Patient: Oh.
Doctor: OK?

A little later in the same exchange, Luca is still confused about the medication and the doctor clarifies the information again:

Doctor: Have you got some Panadol at home?
Patient: Yes I have. Yes, yes, yes.
Doctor: So keep taking them.
Patient: OK. Every two hours?
Doctor: Every four hours.
Patient: Every four hours.
Doctor: Two tablets every four hours.

Towards the end of the exchange, the doctor checks a second time that Luca has understood:

Doctor: Now, d'you understand everything I told you?
Patient: Yeah, yeah. Panadol every four hours.
Doctor: Yeah. Until the pain gets better. Yeah.

Getting patients to express their treatment instructions in their own words is one of the most effective strategies for building shared knowledge and ensuring patient understanding of their diagnosis and treatment.

5.2.6   *Signpost the Hospital Process*

While a large proportion of the activities in the emergency department are concerned with diagnosing and treating a patient's medical ailment (i.e. about the patient's illness), another significant focus is managing the patient through the hospital system, and keeping them informed about what is happening. Doctors and nurses take responsibility for different aspects of this work through their communication with patients.

Most patients feel anxious, disoriented and confused by what's happening to them in the emergency department. While clinicians often do explain the emergency department processes, patients do not always fully grasp or retain this information. Clinicians can help by setting out clearly the steps the patient is likely to go through and the different demands that will be made of him/her along the way.

While many patients in our study expressed anxiety about their medical conditions, only some were explicit about their concerns. One way to alleviate these concerns is to give patients a clear explanation about what is happening and what will happen next.

In this example, the triage nurse gives a detailed explanation of what the patient can expect to happen next:

Nurse: Alright, so like I said, Alwyn, I'll send you up to the next window just to give your Medicare details and things. And then one of our doctors is going to call you through the house doctor section today, so they'll bring you through and have a chat to you in one of the rooms and the house doctor will have a look at your knee, OK, if he needs to.

This extract shows a detailed explanation from the doctor to the patient, Dulcie:

Doctor: == No worries, OK. I'll have a quick listen, ah, but basically I think we'll— we'll need to take a chest X-ray, have a look at your chest and see if there's any obvious area uh that's infected. Um and depending on—and I'll take a little ( ) blood see if there's any—any inflammatory response going on with white cells and things like that and make sure your kidneys are going OK.
Patient: Mm mm [papers rustling]
Doctor: Um and then once all that's back, we'll probably do—I'm sure you've done a spirometry before where we get you to puff into the...
Patient: Oh, please darl', no I'm not going to go any further than—I'll never do it.
Doctor: OK, well I'll—I'll ask you to [patient coughs]—I'll ask you to do your best, that's all I can ask for. [patient coughs] And once we've got all those things I'll, [patient coughs] um, I'll see where we're at and, um, and basically make a decision then. Who do you live with, Dulcie? [patient coughs].

It's easy for clinicians to lose sight of just what the patients do not know about hospital procedures. In the following exchange, the consulting doctor gave his elderly female patient very clear information about her medical condition and explained in detail what the treatment process would be, but did not mention that she would need to be admitted to hospital:

Doctor: I would say that you've got a blockage in your oesophagus.
Patient: Yes?
Doctor: In your gullet.
Patient: Yup.
Doctor: And you need to have someone have another look down with a camera. Just probably like they did last time.
Patient: Yes.
Doctor: And because you can't drink, we probably need to do that today.
Patient: Yeah.
Doctor: So I'll speak to one of the stomach doctors and get him to come and talk to you.
Patient: Yes
Doctor: In the meantime, we'll put um a drip in and give you some fluid into the vein.
Patient: Thank you. Do you want me to stay here all day do you?

Much patient anxiety and disorientation can be attributed to lack of understanding of the emergency department process: what the next stage is and when it might happen. The interaction below is an example of both poor information sharing by the clinician about Victor (can't lift legs—? stroke) and a missed opportunity by Victor and his family to rectify this gap:

Doctor: It's something we do recommend to a lot of our patients who don't walk around because if a clot has formed in your leg then we need to get you Warfarin, a very powerful drug.
Relative: Yeah, yeah no, OK.
Doctor: So we do recommend it once a day let's say. And um. Alright. Any questions, anything you want == to ask me?
Patient: == No.
Doctor: Good. He's certainly ( )
Relative: Like we're still just going to stay here?
Doctor: No. He needs to come into the hospital.
Relative: Oh you are going to admit him?
Doctor: Yep, yeah for pain control and circulatory vasculatory control as well.
Relative: OK.
Doctor: Get the bowel working and get him up and about.
Relative: OK.
Doctor: You happy with it? Are you happy now?
Relative: Yeah I am.
Doctor: Are you happy with that?

The doctor's opening 'Any questions, anything you want == to ask me'? is not taken up by Victor. The daughter's (F) question 'Like we're still just going to stay here?' illustrates the lack of understanding about where Victor would go from that point onwards. It is not clear whether her use of the word 'here' meant the emergency department or the hospital. The registrar assumed she meant the emergency department, hence responded with a 'No' saying Victor would need to come into the hospital. Victor's daughter then used the more formal wording 'admit', which was the first time she had fully understood the next steps. The registrar then provided some additional information as to why. 'Get the bowel working and get him up and about.' The daughter then relinquishes the opportunity to seek further clarification from the doctor after his speedy questions 'You happy with it? Are you happy now'? However, she was initially surprised by the doctor's statement that they would bring Victor into the hospital.

5.2.7   Negotiate Shared Decision-Making About Treatment

Earlier, we argued that effective communication recognises the patient's agency in the interaction. If clinicians have allowed space to the patient to tell their story, have found out what the patient knows and have ensured the medical information has been communicated clearly, then they are likely to have already put the patient in a relatively empowered position. The next step—usually reached during the last activity stage, final medical consultation: diagnosis, treatment and disposition—could be to include the patient in decisions about treatment. As Cordella (2004) noted, if the patient disagrees with the recommended treatment plan, it is likely that they will attempt to renegotiate or refuse to comply.

However, in our data, we have little evidence of patients being given the space to negotiate recommended treatment plans. Possible reasons for this include the patient's lack of familiarity with the consulting doctor, the patient's limited information about his/her medical condition or about other options, and the intimidating nature and experience of the emergency department itself. Yet, even in this context, we would argue that it is important that patients be able to debate, clarify and discuss their treatment options.

In our data, patients do ask questions if they are unclear about their diagnosis and treatment but generally they do not debate or question the doctors' advice.

In the following example, we see Nola (PR bleeding), make a tentative protest about the doctor's recommendation that she have a colonoscopy, but she does not challenge his plan:

D3: And then once it's all settled down we, um, will do…plan another colonoscopy. [Patient is silent. Doctor is shuffling papers.] How does that sound?
Patient: I'd rather have anything else but a colonoscopy.
D3: Well, I'm afraid you've just bought yourself another one.
Patient: [Chuckles]

Despite the momentum of medical efficiency in the emergency department, some patients do succeed in being active in their conversations with clinicians. These are the patients who are able to assert their own agency, usually in interactions with a cooperative clinician.

In Table 5.4, we see that in the more effective example an experienced registrar allows room for Chaitali (PV bleeding) to make an informed health choice. The registrar's question to Chaitali about her options immediately builds on their previously shared knowledge, and gives Chaitali the space to make a choice. This is made possible through their already established relationship—which is rare between clinicians and patients in the emergency department and, arguably, occurred because of the patient's palliative care situation. Although there was little room for negotiation because of the critical nature of the patient's condition, the registrar was able to be firm about her limited choice and went on to explain why other options would not be as good. This contrasts with the junior doctor's disposition in the less effective example we presented in Chap. 4, where no explanation of treatment was given to Clement, an 84-year-old male who presented with left-sided chest pains.

Table 5.4 Contrasting more and less effective ways to allow the patient to make an informed decision

More effective	Less effective
Doctor: Yeah. So I'll see you again tomorrow. If the bleeding settles down with the tranexamic acid, we'll leave it as it is, OK, and we'll let you go. But if the bleeding continues to increase, then we'll consider doing something else. OK. Really, what are the options? Well you really have to the definitive option. The definitive option is the radiotherapy. *Patient: Oh my God.* *Doctor: OK? So the other thing that we can do is with packing. You had radiotherapy, if I start putting things up, you'll be really, really sore. You understand what I mean?* *Patient: Uh huh* *Doctor: So what they do is normally put a lot of packs, you know, cotton packs in the vagina so as to slow down the bleeding, OK. But if I start doing it now, particularly when you've just had radiotherapy, you're going to be really sore in the bottom.* *Patient: OK.* *Doctor: So do you understand what I mean?* *Patient: Yes.* *Doctor: I'd rather leave you alone, start with the tablets and see whether the things settle down.* *Patient: Yes.* *Doctor: And then, um, just watch you overnight. We've already matched your blood should you suddenly have a big bleed, we can give you some blood. OK. But apart from that, we're not going to do anything extra. OK, just watch you overnight here.* *Patient: Yeah. Is it OK to take this tranexamic acid like this? Is it OK?* *Doctor: You're bleeding, of course ( ).* *Patient: I know, I know, I'm…yeah, yeah.* *Doctor: Yeah. You know, anything to stop the bleeding. Because you are coming in a hospital, all relating to bleeding.* *Patient: I know.* *Doctor: Tranexamic acid has this problem, OK, it can form clots. OK.* *Patient: Yeah.* *Doctor: And you start clotting in an unusual spot of course, you know,* *Patient: == Yes ==*	*Dr: I give you good news or bad news?* *Patient: Alright.* *Dr: Which one?* *Patient: Bad one first.* *Dr: Bad one first. OK you did a scan and we found some clots. Multiple. Several clots in the chest. Right that's the bad news. The good news, we found out why you have clots It's not from the heart. The heart's not going to fail.* *Patient: OK*

Table 5.4 (continued)

More effective	Less effective
In this example, the oncology registrar calls on his knowledge shared with Chaitali (PV bleeding), accepts Chaitali's choice—'That's fine', and allows the patient to make the final decision about her treatment 'OK, that's not a problem. So you ( ) are the boss I say. == I have no problem with that'. *Doctor: == we don't want it. But from home when you're bleeding, I mean of course we don't want you to bleed to death. Whereas the potential side effects hasn't happened yet. You know, we've got to treat what's obvious and the obvious thing is bleeding. OK. Now, remember how the last time we [ ] you just wanted oral chemotherapy. Is that right? You know, you didn't want to have the injection, the carboplatin?* *Patient: Yeah.* *Doctor: Have you had a thought, and have you…* *Patient: Yes, I thought I'm going to [go] with the tablet.* *Doctor: You want to go to with the tablets, OK. That's fine.* *Patient: I don't think I can stand this chemo.* *Doctor: OK, that's not a problem. So you ( ) are the boss I say. == I have no problem with that*	*In this example above, the junior doctor delivered the 'good news, bad news' item after Clement (chest pain) had been in the acute section of an emergency department for 7 hrs. The junior doctor wanted to give the feedback to the patient before he left for the day at the end of his shift. It is clear that the time pressure of the shift ending, the late delivery of the diagnostic information to the doctor and the difficulties with English have resulted in a diagnosis with little finesse, given the gravity of the situation. The junior doctor's 'good news, bad news' was preceded by Clement asking the doctor to give him 'the bad news' earlier in the consultation. Thus, the junior doctor did take his cue from Clement. Cross-cultural differences and novice practice affected the quality and comprehensibility of the delivery of diagnosis*

5.2.8 Repeat, Check and Clarify Throughout

Patients can be overwhelmed by information and it can be difficult for them to register the different levels of importance of what they are being told or asked. Repeating key information is a way to check and confirm that patients have understood. Repeating questions is a way of ensuring that all clinicians involved in a patient's care understand the problem. These practices are more relevant when patients are elderly, distressed or do not have English as a first language.

In the following example a junior doctor, who also did not have English as her first language, carefully repeats information a couple of times about what has happened and how long the injury will take to heal. Ghadir (back pain) also had English as her second language:

Doctor: When you fell down onto that bone, it's called a coccyx point, the coccyx… bone. It's a very thin area…and when you fell down on to there…it's going to be sore…but most likely you don't need to do anything done for it.

Doctor: That needs to take time…to get better. The bruising is going to be…the…the pain itself…probably at least for one…one week.

Doctor: When you fell directly into that area, the bruising of the bone is probably one of the worst you can get. Very, very sore. It's going to be a bit prolonger than normal bruising on your arm or anywhere else.

Doctor: So it's going to be a pro…a painful part of that area for at least a week.

In the following example, the nurse reinforces the doctor's instructions and offers reassurance:

Nurse: So when are you—are you coming back again? Or going to the GP?
Patient: Yeah, no, the other—that doctor said that—just to go to the GP in about three days ==
Nurse: == OK. That's good. If you're at all worried you can come back soon, you can come back here or anything like that.

5.3   Conclusion

In this chapter, we have focused on communicating medical knowledge and have detailed communicative strategies that can be used to communicate medical information effectively. However, these present only one side of the communication process—that of communicating information. Just as central to effective communication is the interpersonal relationship—that is, establishing and maintaining the relationship between the clinician and patient. We identify two strong rationales for clinicians to build an interpersonal connection. Firstly, the interpersonal aspects of the communication between clinicians and patients help to personalise medical knowledge, making it relevant to individual patients, which in turn makes it more likely that patients will understand it. Secondly, building relationships with patients also promotes the patient's agency through a process of collaborative knowledge-building and shared decision-making. This makes it more likely that patients will comply with treatment and advice.

In the next chapter, we argue that in order to improve the effectiveness of the medical care that is delivered, clinicians must find more accessible and patient-centred ways to communicate medical information and they must establish a more individual, 'human' connection with patients. In that chapter, we also detail specific communication strategies that emergency clinicians can use to enhance the interpersonal dimensions of their care.

References

Buckley, B., McCarthy, D., Forth, V., Tanabe, P., Schmidt, M., Adams, J., & Engel, K. (2013). Patient input into the development and enhancement of emergency department discharge instructions: A focus group study. *Journal of Emergency Nursing, 39*(6), 553–561.

Cordella, M. (2004). *The dynamic consultation: a discourse analytical study of doctor–patient communication*. Amsterdam: John Benjamins.

Mishler, E. G. (1984). *The discourse of medicine: Dialectics of medical interviews*. New Jersey: Ablex Publishing Corporation.

Chapter 6
Effective Clinician–Patient Communication: Strategies for Bridging the Interpersonal Gap

6.1 Introduction

A key finding of our study is that establishing a positive interpersonal relationship with the patient has implications beyond making the patient 'feel good' about his or her experience in the emergency department. The evidence we have from the many recorded interactions is that positive interpersonal relationships between clinicians and patients result in a higher degree of patient involvement, which in turn produce better clinical outcomes, such as mutually agreed treatment plans and better patient compliance.

Rapport and empathy are integral to the development of interpersonal relationships between clinicians and patients, and are central to the effective implementation of patient-centred care. Empathy means being able to imagine and share another's subjective experience. In the clinical context, Brock and Salinsky (1993) define empathy as 'the skills used to decipher and respond to the thoughts and feelings passing from the patient to the physician'. By giving patients agency (power) in the process, clinicians help patients become involved and gain a sense of control over their own healthcare. Reassuring patients, alleviating their anxiety and acknowledging their personal experiences of illness and injury are other ways in which clinicians can make the emergency department experience a more positive one. These are all aspects of patient-centred care which can only be realised through patient-centred communication.

In this chapter we detail specific communication strategies that emergency clinicians can use to enhance the interpersonal dimensions of their care. These strategies include introducing themselves to patients and explaining their roles, addressing the patient by their first name, using informal and colloquial language, giving supportive feedback, valuing the patient's concerns, initiating and responding to interpersonal chat and using humour and laughter, and demonstrating cultural sensitivity. These strategies are derived from the audio-recordings of patient–clinician interac-

© Springer-Verlag Berlin Heidelberg 2015   125
D. Slade et al., *Communicating in Hospital Emergency Departments,*
DOI 10.1007/978-3-662-46021-4_6

tions over the course of 82 patient journeys through the emergency department from the point of triage to disposition.

Factors that can challenge the development of rapport and empathy between patients and clinicians in emergency departments include severe constraints on the time that clinicians have face-to-face with patients; the lack of pre-established relationships between patients and clinicians; and the short-term and episodic nature of emergency department care. These challenges can be overcome. Indeed, our analyses demonstrated that a key contributor to the development of effective interpersonal relationships between emergency department clinicians and patients was the *willingness* of the doctor or nurse to engage with the patient on an interpersonal level and to open up their interactions with patients to encourage their participation and involvement in their care. As many of our examples of actual clinician–patient consultations show, an accurate diagnosis often took much longer to attain if the patient did not feel like an active participant in the interaction. These interpersonal strategies need to operate simultaneously with the strategies outlined in the previous chapter.

Doctors and nurses are generally perceived as experts in health care. Patients are therefore sometimes less inclined to assert or involve themselves in healthcare decisions. To encourage patients to take a more active role, it is the clinicians who need to reduce the professional distance between themselves and patients. In our study, we observed clinicians who did this effectively by using the strategies we have listed above, and detail below—for example, addressing the patient by their first name, using informal and colloquial language, giving supportive feedback and valuing the patient's concerns. According to our data, when clinicians incorporated these interpersonal strategies into their medical expertise and practice, patients' subjective experiences of the emergency department were affected in a much more positive way.

Before we describe the patient-centred communication strategies clinicians can use to develop rapport and empathy, we provide an example that shows a failure to attend to the patient's interpersonal needs.

In the following lengthy extract, we see a repeated lack of empathy and rapport, or acknowledgement of the patient's pain, by the clinical staff. This first exchange is between Natasha (post-op infection due to a breast augmentation) and the triage nurse:

N: And what brings you into the hospital?
Patient: Bloody agonising—agonising pain. I had a breast aug ... I had a breast augmentation three weeks ago.
N: Yes.
Patient: And I felt pains in my chest. I think they are a normal part of the = = ( ).
N: OK.
Patient: And then today I started to really feel unwell and I feel like it's a heart attack actually. Just really sharp pains in my chest and my left breast is swollen () fever, gone down my arm, you know ...

The nurse concentrates on details of the medical condition, providing no recognition of the patient's repeated expressions of pain:

N: OK, so it's particularly the left one.
Patient: It's the = = right one ...
N: And = = () swollen, or ...
Patient: Yep, yep, and that's where all the pain is.
N: OK. And how long has that been like that for?
Patient: The pain has been since I had the op, but it's ...
N: OK, but the swelling and the ...
Patient: Probably since early this evening, this afternoon.
N: So it's just today that it's come?
Relative: Well no, you've had pain for a while.
Patient: I've had pain and it's got progressively worse but the real temperature and the agonising pain was tonight, today.
N: And sorry, you said three weeks ago?
Patient: Three weeks ago, yup.
N: You had it done, OK. And have you had a follow-up appointment or anything?
Patient: I have, yes, I did.
N: Yes. When was that?
Patient: When did I have that? Last week? It was fine.

When the patient said:

Patient: I actually am in such pain, I can't tell you.

the nurse still offered no words of comfort.

N: It looks, yeah, it looks bigger than that one.

And this continued:

Patient: Very sore, even that is killing me.
N: Yeah.

Although the nurse did attempt to reassure the patient by explaining that such infections were relatively common and could be treated easily she did not show empathy for the patient's pain and extreme discomfort.

N: = = Yeah, look, you know, they are—they are relatively common. Um, and it's— you know, it's not due, not due to anything, such as hygiene or anything like that. It just happens sometimes. And certainly not remarkable, but easily treated most of the time.

The nurse's later comments to a fellow nurse seemed to sum up her approach to the case:

N: I think—I think it might be alright. She seemed quite—she's got a—she had a boob job done () got infected.

After a 3-hour wait, the patient was seen by a (male) doctor. The patient was concerned, as she had been with the triage nurse, to highlight her pain. However, the
doctor proceeds with factual questions:

Doctor: Right. So what happened? You had the operation and …
Patient: And I've just been in terrible pain.
Doctor: Only on the left side?
Patient: On the left side, yeah.

The doctor then asked a series of specific questions:

Doctor: Any discharge from the area? Right. It's not oozing? It's got no oozing?

When the patient described her pain explicitly, the doctor did not pick up on this but
rather went straight onto asking about her temperature:

Patient: But it's definitely an infection I'm in agony and it's there, and just down
    my arm…
Doctor: Have you had temperature = = () and all of that?
Patient: = = Yeah, my temperature is high, yeah. Absolutely.
Doctor: So the operation was about three weeks ago? = =
Patient: = = Three weeks ago.
Doctor: Who did it?

The doctor then examined the patient, and continued questioning her in order to
establish a diagnosis, and begin the process of treatment. The doctor prescribed
medication to bring the patient's temperature down, but did not mention her pain.
Even when the patient reminded him about the pain, the doctor did not respond
empathetically:

Doctor: And no allergies, any medications or anything? OK. Let's have a look at it.
    We'll give you something in a minute to bring the temperature down.
Patient: And the pain.
Doctor: Yeah. What sort of thing did they give you for pain normally?

It was only when the patient cried out in pain following an injection that the doctor made his first interpersonal gesture; however, the focus quickly returned to the
medical:

Doctor: I'm putting in a drip so we can give you some access, that will give you the
    pain relief through that, we take the bloods through that as well. Just a sharp (),
    going one, two, three.
Patient: Oh. Jesus Christ. Ow, ow.
Doctor: Sorry.
Patient: Ow. Ow.
Doctor: Sorry. Oh, that's fine, that's the worst bit. You haven't been vomiting have
    you?

Throughout the patient's emergency department care no doctor or nurse expressed
sympathy for her pain or anxiety. By simply validating the patient's concern and

providing supportive feedback (two of the strategies outlined below) the quality of the patient experience would have been immeasurably improved.

6.2 Bridging the Interpersonal Gap—Effective Strategies for Developing Rapport and Empathy with Patients

Table 6.1 outlines the communication strategies that clinicians can employ to develop rapport and empathy with the patient, and gives examples from the audio-recorded transcripts. These interpersonal strategies complement the communication strategies used to communicate medical information effectively (outlined in Chap 5). In the following sections we take each of these communication strategies and provide examples.

6.2.1 Introduce Yourselves as Clinicians and Explain your Roles

Throughout patient-centred communication literature, including patient satisfaction surveys (such as the NSW Health Patient Survey 2008), patients consistently stated that when clinicians introduced themselves and explained their role, it helped alleviate their anxieties. One of the recommendations of the Garling Inquiry (Garling 2008) was that clinicians wear name and position badges at all times. Apart from needing to feel reassured in what can be a bewildering context, patients also need to know who is questioning them and to what end, if they are to cooperate fully with the process. Our data showed that while clinicians regularly introduce themselves to patients, they frequently do not specify their status or their role in the emergency department.

Patients have encounters with many people, not all of them clinicians, during their stay in the emergency department. For example, one patient we recorded, Nola, had 172 different encounters during the time that she was in the emergency department. This meant that every 29 secs either she engaged with someone or the consultation was interrupted. Add to this the fact that Nola was an elderly patient who was in pain, and the potential for confusion is increased.

In Nola's initial medical consultation, the junior doctor did not introduce herself. The nurse (N2), who was doing her 'obs', announced the doctor's arrival (N2 'The doctor'll ask you questions now') but Nola did not register the information and thought the junior doctor was 'a nurse'. This assumption may well have affected the kind of information that Nola provided. After responding to many questions about her medical history Nola finally expressed her confusion by asking the doctor:

Nola: So what's it … what are you taking all the info for? There was another little girl that's gonna take a lot of info.
Doctor: There are lots of people you'll be talking to. I'm the doctor … I'm one of the doctors who'll be looking after you.
Nola: Oh … you're a doctor. I'm really sorry I thought you were … just a nurse…

Table 6.1 Strategies for developing rapport and empathy with patients

Communication strategy	Description	Examples from authentic recorded interactions
1. Introduce yourself and describe your role	Alleviate patient anxiety by introducing yourself and explaining your role in order to clearly establish your medical expertise	'Good morning. My name's () and I'm one of the surgical registrars here. I work with Dr (). He told me you were coming in.'
2. Use inclusive language	Put patients at ease and create an atmosphere where the patient feels more included in the decision-making process by using the patient's name and the pronoun 'we'	'We'll get you through as soon as we can, George. We're just going to have another look down your throat with a camera, and because you can't drink, we probably need to do that today.'
3. Use colloquial language and softening expressions to put patients at ease	Minimise the strangeness of the emergency department context by using colloquial language	'Have you noticed any blood from your bottom at all?' 'Just pop up on there for me.'
	Soften commands and requirements of the patient with expressions of probability, e.g. I think, probably	'And because you can't drink, we probably need to do that today.' 'With that low a blood count and with your history of heart attacks, I think it's very likely that we need to transfuse you.'
4. Give positive, supportive feedback	Validating the patient's concerns by expressing empathy and alleviating patient anxiety by showing interest, approval and engagement with the patient	Patient: 'I'd say it's probably about a month, probably about—I had a haemorrhoid.' Doctor: 'Yeah.' Patient: 'And I had that lanced a couple of weeks ago.' Doctor: 'Yeah.' Patient: 'And, um …' Doctor: 'I'm feeling for you.'
	Mirror patients' comments regarding symptoms, attitudes or concerns	Patient: 'They were really big clots like that.' Doctor: 'Yeah, so really big clots.'
	Express personal attitudes and values to show support	'Because you are absolutely right. I don't blame you. I don't blame you. But you've done all the right things.'
5. Recognise the patient's perspective	Validating the patient's concerns by expressing a positive attitude to the patient's thoughts and feelings about their medical conditions or their responses to treatment	'No. You're not going crazy. I can appreciate how uncomfortable it must feel. It's not a very nice test.'

Table 6.1 (continued)

Communication strategy	Description	Examples from authentic recorded interactions
6. Intersperse medical talk with interpersonal chat	Put patients at ease and reduce the professional distance between you by chatting to them about aspects of life that are unrelated to their medical conditions	'You play Rugby Union do you? So who do you think is going to win the World Cup this year?'
7. Share laughter and jokes	Alleviate anxiety and lighten the atmosphere by sharing jokes and laughter that express solidarity and inclusiveness	'You've got to have another needle, have you? Ooh! You're the lucky one!'
8. Demonstrate intercultural sensitivity	Elicit and listen to details of a patient's cultural background and don't make cultural generalisations or assumptions based on cultural stereotypes	N1 'How long have you been in [XX city]?' P 'About 7, 8 years?' ——- N1 'So country of birth, where were you born?' F [European country]

At the conclusion of the initial medical consultation, the junior doctor announced that she was waiting on the results of tests and would return in due course. Again Nola tried to connect with the identity of the junior doctor:

Doctor: It can take just a little while to get the results, but I'll come back and let you know.
Nola: Right. Thank you doctor. Doctor who?
Doctor: (laughs)
Nola: Yes. What's ... what's your name?
Doctor: [Name]
Nola: [Name]. Nice name.

By contrast, in another emergency department, Jack (feeling unwell, weak), was in a wheelchair and in the advanced stages of multiple sclerosis. He had arrived at 9 am and was first seen by the doctor at 1.05 pm. The junior doctor, who must have known that Jack had had a long wait, was particularly welcoming to the patient:

Doctor: So you're Jack, that's right?
Patient: I'm Jack, yeah.
Doctor: Ah, hi Jack. Nice to meet you. [D1 shakes patient's hand]
Patient: How are you?

Below are examples of how other doctors and nurses introduce themselves:
   One of the doctors in the 'fast track' section of one emergency department was particularly welcoming to a young patient who had severely lacerated his thumb

and who was in great pain. The senior doctor was mentoring a young student doctor throughout the consultation and greeted the patient:

Dcotor: Hi, g'day. G'day I'm [Dr X], I'm one of the emergency doctors. How are you feeling right now?

In another emergency department, Ghadir (back pain) was anxious to know the level of experience of the doctor who had attended to her. She had just been told that the medication she would be on would not interfere with her breast milk and felt uncertain about this and about her diagnosis. Ghadir's husband also commented on the couple's ignorance about the junior doctor's experience and status and how this would affect their trust of the diagnosis and treatment:

Husband: [ ]. (Don't know if) she [referring to the doctor] is provisional one or ...?
Researcher: Yeah.
Husband: Or a new one or ...?
Researcher: That's interesting isn't it?
Husband: How can I trust ...?
Researcher: Yeah, you don't—you don't feel comfortable because you don't know ...
Husband: Yeah, I don't know who I am talking to.
Researcher: ... her level.
Husband: Yes.
Researcher: Yeah. That's interesting, isn't it? They don't wear badges or ...
Husband: They should, absolutely...

As the above interchange between the researcher and Ghadir's husband illustrates, a clinician's failure to introduce themselves or their role can jeopardise the establishment of trust and confidence between clinicians and patients. This may lead to lack of agreement in terms of treatment plans and potentially noncompliance with recommended treatment.

6.2.2   Use Inclusive Language

When clinicians use inclusive language, they help put patients at ease in the interaction and create an environment where the patient feels more included in making decisions. Effective inclusive language techniques include using the patient's first name and using the inclusive pronoun 'we' to include the patient in the actions and decisions of the clinical staff. Using the patient's first name allows patients to feel personally identified in what can be a very intimidating environment. In the following example, one clinician addresses Mara (blockage of oesophagus) by her first name:

Nurse: So, Mara, your blood pressure is a bit high so you've probably not kept your tablets down.

With Wilson (sore toe) the nurse focused very specifically on the patient's statements about how long he had waited to get into the emergency department and encouraged him by saying it had not in fact been all that long given the current deteriorating situation. She used his name and positive feedback to try to soften the blow of his long waiting time:

Nurse: Oh, that's pretty good. If you'd been half an hour later you should see the patients in the corridor now. Now Wilson, are you allergic to anything?
Wilson: No.
Nurse: OK. And what medications == are you on?

The use of first names has the effect of putting the patient at ease in the interaction and helps create an environment where the patient feels more included in the process. Some clinicians, more typically nurses, use terms of endearment as a way of making patients feel included, although these may be interpreted as patronising, particularly when used with elderly patients. The nurse with Nola (PR bleeding), tried to encourage her to co-operate in this way:

Nurse: Yeah, I'll put all those in too for you. That's a girl.
Nola: Um I probably, I don't know, but it's on the cards that I could ...
Nurse: OK, I'll just == put a thing on.
Nola: == bleed again...
Nurse: Don't worry. I'll put a thing on. There you go, gorgeous. Just pop up on there for me.

Other examples from our data included:

Nurse: OK, darling. I'm just going to leave that on your arm.:
Admissions Clerk: I need to check your details, darling. Um, are you a [street]? And is that [suburb]?
Nurse: Here, pop this over, darling, hold it down a bit.
Nurse: Do you have oxygen at home, darlin'? Do you have puffers?
Nurse: Have you got an armband on, darling?
Nurse: Do you want a mask or are you happy holding a pipe, darl?
Nurse: OK. How about that pain at the moment, honey?

The inclusive pronoun 'we' can be used to co-opt the patient into the healthcare team. With Graydon (cardiology admission), the nurses emphasised the team nature of their work, by alternating their turns in the talk, by using 'we', and by explaining what the other person was about to do. In this way, the nursing staff succeeded in recruiting Graydon as a team participant, while emphasising the patient's role as an active agent in the consultation:

Nurse 1: We're going to count to six. No chest pain at all?
Graydon: No, not at the moment. No.
Nurse 2: Good.
Nurse 1: Right. So [Nurse 2] is going to put a cannula in and take some bloods now.
Nurse 2: How do they usually go taking blood from you?
Nurse 1: We're pretty much done here.
Nurse 2: OK. Yeah.

Nurse 1: Do you have any allergies? Oh, you've got an armband. Right. There's some stickers for you [N3]. I'll go and get this ECG on.

Nurse 2: OK. Just give your hand a bit of a pump for me. And hold it. Have a little poke round there OK? Just give a nice, cold swab. Stay nice and still for me …

Clinicians also used 'we' when referring to the medical procedures that would take place in the emergency department. This reinforced the fact that the medical care that Donna (anal fissure), was receiving was a team effort. Nurses admitting patients frequently work in pairs and in the example below, nurse 2 and nurse 3 were settling Donna and changing her into her gown. Nurse 2 goes back and forth between offering her assistance both personally and institutionally (collectively):

Nurse 1: Just lie on—maybe lie on your side rather than = = [two nurses working together, Nurse 1 and Nurse 2]

Nurse 2: Yeah.

Nurse 1: = =sitting on it. Do you find lying down on your side might be a bit more comfortable for you?

Donna: Yeah, yeah I just = =, yeah.

Nurse 1: = =What we'll do is we'll get you into a um, an actual gown, here's one, here we are—

Donna: Yeah.

Nurse 1: –there's one here, opens up at the back, and I'll get you to lie down and, um yeah, we'll come back, I'll come back to you in a minute OK? Alright just try and = =

The use of 'we' draws in the patient as an active agent in the consultation, juxtaposed with the use of 'I' when the doctor's professional expertise is foregrounded. We see this with Luca (stiff neck):

Nurse: We'll get you through as soon as we can, Luca.

6.2.3   Use Colloquial Language and Softening Expressions

When presenting or requesting medical information, most clinicians are careful to recast their technical terms in more everyday and sometimes quite colloquial terms, so that their patients can understand what they are saying:

Doctor: Have you noticed any blood from your bottom at all?

The use of these everyday words not only ensures comprehension but also helps to put patients at ease in what is in reality a very formal and unfamiliar context. The registrar with David (sore testes) uses the same technique:

Doctor: What we do have there is what we call epididymo-orchitis. That's just our fancy way of saying infection.

The strangeness of the emergency department context, and the patient's relative disempowerment within it, can also be minimised by the use of two common 'softening' expressions:

- *just* or *only* to mitigate commands
- expressions of probability rather than certainty to temper statements, e.g. probably, I think.

These expressions—examples of modality and modulation—are language features that make statements less definite, or introduce an element of possibility. Examples include just, may, might, perhaps, can, would, should, I think, probably. By using this language, a space is created for another view, belief or opinion which allows for disagreement by the other person involved in the interaction. The modulation of statements and questions has the effect of tempering the directness of what is said to patients and can help to mitigate the 'medical' experience for them. Nurses in particular use the mitigating word 'just' frequently, to soften what are in effect commands with which patients need to comply. There are a number of examples in the interaction between Nola (PR bleeding) and the nurse in charge of her admission. Notice how the nurse also uses a colloquial term of endearment (love) and everyday vocabulary (pop up) to make her request ('Get up on the bed now') sound friendly and polite:

Nurse: And just put one arm in, love, only because I'll need to take the other one out anyway, and I'll just get you to pop up on the bed now. Just put that in there. And leave that one out and just pop yourself up there.

Another way of softening the effect of obligations on the patient is for the clinician to phrase them as not completely certain. In the following example we see one of the junior registrars explaining the next steps to Mara (oesophagus blockage). Mara was required to endure further tests, but the doctor softened the blow with several expressions of probability as well as one mitigating *just*:

Doctor: And you need to have someone have another look down with a camera. Just probably like they did last time.
Mara: Yes.
Doctor: And because you can't drink, we probably need to do that today.
Mara: Yeah.
Doctor: Going to have to put, try, I think to put a drip into you.
Mara: Mmhm.
Doctor: With that low a blood count and with your history of heart attacks, I think it's very likely that we need to transfuse you.

The doctor in charge of Jean (review of suture after leg injury) tempered her explanations with both '*just*' and the modality '*probably*':

Doctor: OK. So what we need, just to put a new dressing on.
Mara: Yeah.
Doctor: OK, probably not that thick.

The nurse in the following example also made a technically unnecessary—but re-spect-building—request for the patient's permission:

Nurse: Now I might just move this so that I don't dribble saline on that leg ... OK.
   I'll just wash my hands, if that's OK?

6.2.4   Give Positive and Supportive Feedback

Clinicians can establish positive relationships by using feedback cues that express support for the patient. These cues include evaluative expressions such as *excellent, good, great, that's terrific, well done*, exclamations of surprise and support (e.g. *Wow! Fancy that!*), open questions that encourage the patient to say more and mirroring of the patient's comments, which both implies support and invites further comment. Clinicians often repeat what patients say as a way of checking the information, but this strategy is also a useful way of demonstrating the clinician's valida-tion of the patient's interpersonal experience. These strategies are important ways of validating the patient's concerns by expressing empathy and alleviating patient anxiety by showing interest, approval and engagement with the patient.

In the example below, the triage nurse established rapport with the patient by making it clear that the patient's contributions were an important part of the assess-ment process. In the more effective example, with Mara (blockage of oesophagus) we see evidence of reassuring feedback:

Mara: ... Years ago I was knocked over by a car and I was here for six weeks.
Nurse: Oh my goodness, you've been very lucky.
Nurse: I'll just pop you in the waiting room just now and I'll go and get a bed and
   we'll pop you through.
Mara: Thank you, darling.
Nurse: My pleasure.
Mara: You've been very kind.

In this example, the triage nurse gave reassuring feedback and showed empathy by commenting on Mara's good luck. Even patients like Mara, who arrived at the emergency department with a medical condition that was not necessarily life threat-ening, responded well to these overtures.

Doctors generally maintain a greater professional distance from patients than nurses do. Doctors provide patients with supportive, empathetic and reassuring feedback. However, their responses tend to be more measured. Nurses are more directly involved with managing patients within the hospital system and are less concerned with gathering information about the medical aspects of the case. Poten-tially they have a better opportunity to establish more personal relationships with patients. Expressing support and empathy through feedback is one way they do this. The nurse with Jean (review of suture after leg injury), interacted with the patient in this way. Jean responded positively to the nurse's more personal engagement and re-told the story of her accident in more vivid detail than she had used with the doctor. She also added a commentary about the way it had affected her, which she did not share with the doctor. It was the nurse's enthusiastic responses to Jean's tale that encouraged her to speculate about what had happened, and gave her the opportunity to share her experience:

Nurse: How did it happen?
Jean: [Laughs]
Nurse: You've probably told that many times.
Jean: But it's such a freak thing. I ... like I was walking the dog in the park, it's just ridiculous, and I stood on a stick, I must have, I stood on a stick with this foot and it's come up in the air and gone into this leg.
Nurse: Whoa!
Jean: But I had long pants on and I cannot understand. So I didn't think ... it didn't tear my pants ...
Nurse: Wow!
Jean: and whether it came up the leg of it ... I ... I don't know that cause = =
Nurse: = = But that's from a stick?
Husband: Mmm!
Jean: Stick!
Nurse: Wow!
Jean: So ... and all I ... because all the blood just came rushing out 'cause it was quite deep, and I felt quite sick, I didn't sort of think about that at the time or look for the stick [giggles] ... but I don't remember the stick going up the pants. But my pants aren't torn ... so it must have been a really, really, really sharp stick.
Nurse: It's very strange isn't it?

Although less frequent, doctors did also provide patients with supportive, empathetic and reassuring feedback. Below, with Donna (HX, anal fissure), the junior doctor gave an empathetic response to Donna's less than delicate description of her pain:

Doctor: Yeah. What's your pain like now out of ten?
Donna: Probably about five.
Doctor: OK. Ah.
Donna: I feel like I've got a screwdriver up my backside most of the time.
Doctor: Yeah, ah look it's ghastly. It's one of those things where you know, you ha— there's not much to show for it, but they're dread—you know people have such discomfort it's awful.

In the example below, the doctor reassures Wilson (sore toe) that he had been giving himself the correct treatment:

Wilson: And I soak it with the Dettol and like a warm = = thing.
Doctor: = = Good.
Wilson: Just warm = = and Dettol.
Doctor: = = It's exactly what you should be doing. OK. Alright.
Wilson: Yeah.

In general, however, although doctors did provide patients with supportive, empathetic and reassuring feedback, their responses tended to be more measured, as the following extracts show. In the first example, the doctor gave Jean (review of suture after leg injury) supportive feedback and warned her what to expect when she unwrapped the wound:

Doctor: And it's no new swelling or pain just below here?
Jean: Sorry?
Doctor: No new pain or swelling just down below?
Jean: No.
Doctor: OK. That's good ... Well, it won't look excellent.

The doctor then gave Jean a positive review of her wound, which was cautious but reassuring for Jean to hear:

Jean: But everything's going OK?
Doctor: Absolutely, yes, looks fine. So = =
Jean: = = She did a good job didn't she?
Doctor: Oh, yes. It's—it's () you know, = = (). [Overtalking]
Jean: = = She was very—very good.
Husband: She was only = =
Jean: = = She was very good.
Husband: We're just worried about this little, you know, the flap. See that bit of skin there.
Doctor: = = No, no, no. Everything seems to = = be reliable.

In the extract below Federica (dizziness, sore ear) presented to the emergency department with her medication list. Before her arrival, she had understood the importance of bringing her medication list to the emergency department, so she had cut off the labels from each box of medication and placed them together in a pile. She had done this possibly because English was not her first language and by bringing the bundle of labels in, it was going to be easier for her to communicate these to the doctor. We see how the junior doctor, who also didn't have English as her first language, gave Federica positive feedback about this strategy.

Doctor: And are you taking any medications, usually?
Federica: Yes.
Doctor: Did you bring them? OK.
Male neighbour: [Background coughing]. They're in her bag.
Federica: Yes. Operation cataract.
Doctor: Cataract. Both eyes?
Federica: Just—and before I have ()—out.
Doctor: Ah-hm. So they fixed = = it so ...
Federica: = = only for (), only for ().
Doctor: Ah-hm.
Federica: = = ()].
Male neighbour: = = ().

Federica: In here. [Patient hands over bundle of medication labels]
Doctor: Oh, that's a smart way of ...
Federica: (), the ()?
Doctor: Uh huh.
*Federica: I take one, and two in the morning and one and two in the night. And that
    one for the depression.*

The examples below demonstrate senior doctors providing supportive feedback in
the final medical consultation (the treatment, diagnosis and disposition stage). In
the first example, the senior doctor displays empathy by acknowledging the dread
of the bowel preparation necessary for a colonoscopy felt by Nola (PR bleeding):

*Nola: I would have gone back to Dr—ah, thingo only to—to have another colonos-
    copy, but it's the lead up to it that ...*
Doctor: The bowel prep's terrible isn't it?
Nola: The—no, the—you know the fluids and that, the ...
Doctor: Yeah, the stuff you drink, yeah.
Nola: Oh God!

When patients are suffering from a serious medical condition, as was the case for
Graydon (cardiology admission), the need for reassurance is often heightened, and
a few reassuring words can make a big difference:

Graydon: Do you want me on my back ... or?
Doctor: No, you're just perfect.

A basic way of showing support for what the patient is saying is to mirror the patient's experience. We saw earlier that clinicians often repeat back what patients say
as a way of checking the information, but this strategy can also demonstrate the clinician's validation of the patient's interpersonal experience. The following extracts
demonstrate how this was done with various patients:

Patient: A week—a week ago.
Nurse: One week ago. In this hospital?

———-

Nurse: Did this just start yesterday?
Patient: Two days ago.
Nurse: Two days.

———-

Nurse: Have you had a fever or the shakes or anything?
Patient: Evening time.
Nurse: In the evening time. OK ...

Although many clinicians express empathy for patients' pain, most of the time clinicians do not give feedback that expresses personal attitudes or experiences about
the patient's illness or test results. When clinicians did express thoughts to patients
about their illness, we noticed that this was well received by patients. This female
junior doctor was particularly sympathetic to Donna (HX, anal fissure), disclosing

that her mother had experienced a similar condition. She was thus able to express
personal attitudes and values about Donna's illness and predicament:

*Doctor: Right, alright. I need to have a look at you. I'm going to go and wash my
hands and then I will come back and then I will have a chat to someone and we'll
try and work out = =*
Donna: Yeah.
Doctor: = = what we're going to do next. Poor thing.
Donna: Alright.
Doctor: I feel—I feel bad for you 'cause it's awful.
Donna: It's just—'cause it's = =
Doctor: Yeah.

Here a more senior doctor expresses his positive opinion on the blood pressure results (previously high) for Wilson (sore toe):

Doctor: Is your blood pressure under control now?
Wilson: Yes.
Doctor: What was it?
Wilson: Today was 128.
Doctor: OK, brilliant. Well done. OK
*Wilson: Um, I was ... I saw him about three weeks ago or four weeks ago, it was
115. So the blood pressure's down,*
Doctor: Mm mm ......
Doctor: Are you diabetic?
Wilson: No.
Doctor: Good. Anything else going on? What ... what = = respiratory []?

6.2.5 Recognise the Patient's Perspective

Yet another empathetic strategy is to reassure the patient that they are justified in
feeling worried about their condition. Nola (PR bleeding) was embarrassed by her
symptoms and anxious about what was happening to her. Both the nurse and the
doctor who had responsibility for the initial medical consultation (initial assessment
and stabilisation stage) made an effort to make her feel that her responses were quite
normal:

Nola: Um I probably, I don't know, but it's on the cards that I could ...
Nurse: OK, I'll just = = put a thing on.
Nola: = = bleed again.
Nurse: Don't worry. I'll put a thing on.

———

Doctor: Do you have any allergies?
Nola: Mm? [patient groans with pain].
Doctor: Nola? Do you have any allergies?

Nola: [breathing heavily]. No.
Doctor: You're doing really well.
Nola: I don't think so. I'm a real cocktail when it comes to needles.
Nurse: You're doing well, darl, just stay very still for me.

6.2.6   Intersperse Medical Talk with Interpersonal Chat

Some clinicians seek to put their patients at ease during the consultation by interspersing their medical talk with informal chat. In other words, the clinician would chat to the patient about aspects of either of their lives unrelated to the illness, but usually introduced into the conversation in some way by the patient. Used with care, this strategy can contribute positively to building interpersonal rapport, provided the patient perceives the 'chat' as somehow relevant to them.

In this example, the doctor followed David's (swollen testes) cue during the history-taking, and then pursued a lengthy discussion (not included here) with David about a shared interest, rugby:

Patient: I don't actually have any pain in the knee and it's a total mess. Did all the
*   ligaments, bit more cartilage out in 1960.*
Doctor: Playing football?
Patient: Yes.
Doctor: What kind of football?
Patient: Rugby Union.
Doctor: Rugby Union?
Patient: Yeah.
Doctor: So what do you reckon is going to happen in the World Cup?

Demonstrating an interest in the patient's experiences outside the emergency department is another way of creating rapport and a human connection. In the extract below, a triage nurse asks the patient, who has just returned from Victoria, about bushfires that had been widely publicised at the time.

Nurse: Um, have you—were you actually involved in the bushfires?
Patient: No, no.
Nurse: OK.
Patient: My son had a friend, he and his wife, you know, died in a car, but I mean um
Nurse: Yeah.
Patient: That was sad but that—that wasn't the reason.
Nurse: It's tough isn't it?
Patient: Oh it was awful.
Nurse: Particularly when we [city] went through that.

Relevant and constrained personal disclosure can also help to express empathy. In the next example, the very empathetic junior doctor went as far as telling the patient that her mother had suffered a similar condition and therefore she understood her predicament more fully:

Patient: = = no joke, just can't put up with the = =
Doctor: Yeah, yeah, yeah.
Patient: = = pain anymore.
Doctor: Yeah, look I know, that's all = = my mum actually had this problem, my mum
*   has [digestive] disease and it was desperate, like it was so awful, so I really = =*
Patient: Well you just = =
Doctor: = = feel for you, 'cause I = =
Patient: = = you know just when it's really bad = =
Doctor: Yeah.

6.2.7   Share Laughter and Jokes

We observed that the judicious use of humour during clinician–patient consultations
seemed to help ease the patient's anxiety. The doctor responsible for the initial medical consultation (assessment and stabilisation stage) for Jean (review of suture after
leg injury), shared a laugh with Jean over the size of the antibiotic capsules which
had been prescribed earlier. This helped to develop the rapport between them:

Doctor: No, no. You just continue with your antibiotics …
Jean: Oh, they're huge ones, you know, like horse tablets [laughs] = = two a day.
Doctor: = = [Laughs] Are they the () dissolvable ones?
Jean: No.

In the following extract, Nola (PR bleeding), made a joke at the expense of the senior nurse. Nola was concerned that her comments might have seemed a little rude
but the nurse showed her good humour and everyone joined in the laughter. Nola
even contributed with humour directed at her own condition:

Nola: = = And it was Dr [specialist's surname], you wouldn't know him.
Doctor: No, I don't.
Nola: He's before your time. This lady might, I doubt it.
Doctor: [Chuckles]
Nola: Up on the corner.
Nurse: Yeah, I'm the old one. [Laughs]
Nola: Dr [says specialist's name] up there on the corner.
Nurse: No, I wouldn't. I have been here that long, but anyway.
Nola: No, I'm not being rude.
Nurse: I know you're not, sweetheart. I'm pulling your leg.
Nola: Oh, no, don't pull it today. [Laughs]
Nurse: [Laughs].

However, some patients commented on the inappropriate use of humour in the emergency department. Here is one particularly insensitive example. This patient had
multiple sclerosis. In finding out how incapacitated he might be, the nurse asked:

Nurse: Now what level down are you?
Patient: Ah, what ...
Nurse: Incapacitated.
Patient: Well I ...
Nurse: I don't know your story, why you're in a wheelchair?
Patient: Oh, MS.
Nurse: MS is it? Oh, OK, right. Fair enough. Didn't get (). I thought you must have
  dived off the pool. Bang, OK? MS!! = =

Humour done sensitively and taking into account the patient's particular context can help ease anxiety and stress and help lessen the distance between the patient and the clinician.

6.2.8   Demonstrate Intercultural Sensitivity

Cross-cultural awareness is a basic requirement for clinicians who are dealing with multicultural populations. In the less effective example in Table 6.2 below, an agency nurse inadvertently revealed her cultural assumptions. Chaitali (PV bleeding), was from a South-East Asian country. Although Chaitali had a strong accent in English, her English was very good. The nurse and the patient were discussing the patient's son.

6.3   Conclusion

In Australia, as in many other places in the world, patients want patient-centred care that explores the main reason for their visit, acknowledges their concerns and satisfies their need for information. These are all central in helping to alleviate anxiety and to reach a timely diagnosis. To achieve this patient-centred care, clinicians need an integrated understanding of the world from the patient's perspective, and an appreciation of the whole person and their emotional needs and life issues (Stewart 2001, p. 445). However, the complexities inherent in emergency care—where multiple patients may need urgent treatment simultaneously—often lead to a prioritisation of medical tasks over the experiences and sensibilities of people involved. Here, so often, interpersonal communication—attending to the interpersonal needs of the patient—comes second to the goal of saving lives and making people well where the dominance of medical concerns overrides the patient's personal circumstances. In critically ill patients this is necessary but with patients not in immediate danger, this prioritisation has implications for both the quality and safety of the patient's experience as discussed in Chap 4.

   In the five hospital emergency departments we studied, we found that often patient stories were not picked up, patients were given few opportunities to contribute, and the dominance of medical questions often overrode the patient's personal

Table 6.2 Contrasting more and less effective ways to demonstrate cultural sensitivity

More effective	Less effective
Nurse: How long have you been in [city]? *Patient: About seven, eight years?* ———- *Nurse: So country of birth, where were you born?* *Relative: [European country]*	Nurse: Yeah. OK, that's OK. Is someone here with you, or are you alone? Patient: Yeah, I'm on my—yeah—yeah—() my son is here actually. He's a lecturer in the university Nurse: Who just—who's the next of kin? Patient: My son Nurse: And what's his first name? Patient: [name] Nurse: How do you spell that? [chuckles] Patient: [patient spells out the name, [name]] Nurse: Where are you from, originally? Malaysia somewhere? Indonesia? Patient: [Says name of country] Nurse: [Repeats name of country]. Oh () on that, OK. What's your son's telephone or is it the same number as yours? Patient: His [number] Nurse: (), OK. And he obviously speaks English, I hope?
In this example, the nurse doing triage chats informally to Marchello (suspected DVT) about where he was born. The triage nurse could tell from his accent that Marchello was not Australian born, and as he was presenting with a sore leg after a long flight, she showed awareness of the fact that he might be new to the city. She did not need to ask his place of birth but in doing so, showed sensitivity and recognition of Marchello's cultural background	In this example, the agency nurse laughed when she heard Chaitali's (PV bleeding) son's name. She bundled a number of South-East Asian countries together to determine Chaitali's country of origin. She misunderstood Chaitali's comment that her son was a lecturer at an Australian university and then questioned Chaitali's son's English proficiency. In the more effective example alongside, N1's question 'Where were you born?' would be far more culturally appropriate than the agency nurse's question

circumstances. Patients were not often encouraged to ask questions, questioning by doctors restricted the range of possible responses and insufficient explanations were provided. In the follow-up interviews we conducted with patients, we found that when satisfied with their emergency department experience, patients always referred to interpersonal aspects of their treatment—such as caring and attentive staff and clinicians who listened to them. Although doctors bring considerable scientific knowledge to bear on diagnostic decisions when treating patients, our evidence-based research has shown that what they obtain from patients themselves is crucial to good diagnostic practice.

In this and the previous chapter we have argued that there are two broad areas of communication which affect the quality and safety of the patient journey through the emergency department:

- how medical knowledge is communicated, and
- how clinician–patient relationships are established and maintained.

Both of these are crucial for effective communication: to deliver care effectively, clinicians must communicate care effectively.

References

Brock, C. D., & Salinsky, J. V. (1993). Empathy: An essential skill for understanding the physician-patient relationship in clinical practice. *Family Medicine, 25,* 245–248.

Garling, P. (2008). Final report of the special commission of inquiry: Acute care services in nsw public hospitals: vols. 1–2. Sydney: Special Commission of Inquiry.

NSW Health Patient Survey (2008). Statewide Report. Sydney: NSW Health. http://www.bhi.nsw.gov.au/_data/assets/pdf_file/0017/212039/Annual_Patient_Survey_Report_2008.pdf.

Stewart, M. (2001). Towards a global definition of patient centred care. *British Medical Journal, 322,* 444–445 (Clinical research ed.).

Chapter 7
Action Strategies for Implementing Change

7.1 Introduction

In this book, we have described how organisational and clinician practices and roles in emergency departments manifest in particular communication patterns and interactive styles between clinicians and patients. The central figure throughout the book is the patient, and the central question we have asked is: How does communication in emergency departments affect both the quality and safety of the patient experience?

But we have also focused on the clinicians. We have described the intense pressure they work under—a result of insufficient funding to emergency departments, rising patient loads, bed block, patients presenting with multiple morbidities, and increasing linguistic and cultural diversity. In such high-stress contexts, inadequate communication has been shown to be a major source of unsafe situations.

Our onsite recordings demonstrated vulnerable points in clinician–patient interactions, which we have called 'potential risk points' (PRP). We have argued that these have the potential to jeopardise patient safety. If communication is effective, it can also be the best way of controlling potential risks.

As we have shown, communication, whether spoken, gestured, written, or electronic, underpins what is done in the emergency department. From handovers to taking blood, giving medication, talking to patients, listening to colleagues, reading computer screens, or doing resuscitations, clinicians are constantly speaking, listening, reading, and writing. The ways in which the communicative, social, and clinical practices work together in the complex context of the emergency department define the overall quality of the experience for patients and the ultimate work satisfaction of clinicians.

We have found that both the quality of patient care and the patient's experience of that care are negatively affected by two interlinking factors:

© Springer-Verlag Berlin Heidelberg 2015
D. Slade et al., *Communicating in Hospital Emergency Departments,*
DOI 10.1007/978-3-662-46021-4_7

- Contextual complexity: The complex, discontinuous, and fragmented nature of emergency department consultations can result in loss of knowledge transfer, inadequate and confusing explanations, and insensitivity to the patient.
- Foregrounding of the medical over the personal: The failure of clinicians to build rapport and create relationships with patients can inhibit a patient's understanding of a diagnosis and compliance with the treatment.

In this chapter, we present seven action strategies to improve communication in emergency departments. Some of these are organisational; some of these are suggesting complementary evidence-based communication research, vital as a basis for implementing systemic recommendations and change.

7.2   Action Strategies

7.2.1   Achieve a Balance Between Medical and Interpersonal Communication

Our research shows that two broad areas of communication affect the quality of the patient journey through the emergency department: (1) how medical knowledge is communicated and (2) how clinician–patient relationships are established and built. We argue that to deliver care effectively, clinicians must communicate care effectively. To do this, clinicians must build rapport with the patient. We therefore propose that strategies and skills both in communicating medical knowledge and in building interpersonal relationships be a required component in the training and assessment of emergency department clinicians. We summarised and exemplified these communication skills in tables 5.1 and 6.1 and discussed each strategy in detail in Chaps. 5 and 6.

7.2.2   Provide Explicit Explanations to Patients About Processes and Procedures in the Emergency Department

Patients are strangers to the emergency department environment yet they receive very little information about what is going on and what will happen to them. To improve clinician–patient communication, we recommend the following four actions:

Develop an Orientation Protocol Emergency departments should have 'orientation protocols'. This can guide clinicians in conveying both clinical details and process information (such as more general information about the emergency department). Because patients are outsiders to the institutionalised language and patterns of behaviour of emergency department staff, this can lead to anxiety, incomprehension, and interpersonal alienation. While they *are* often given information and explanations about the processes of the emergency department, they often do not understand these fully because they are ill and anxious and because clinicians present the information in complex institutional and medical language.

While we were collecting our data at one of the emergency departments, one of the project nurses introduced a 'green sheet', which included information to help patients understand where they might be in the particular stage of an emergency department consultation. We understand that this initiative was later withdrawn as a result of poor implementation by staff, which led to low use by patients. In principle the idea is an excellent one, because patients are frequently confused and unaware about the timing of processes, which part of the emergency department they are in, or what stage of treatment they are at. The demands on everybody in such a busy environment made the information sheet difficult to implement.

Explain Triage Categories   We recommend that staff tell patients which triage category they have given them, and the expected waiting time.

In some places, for example Hong Kong, patients are usually told their allocated triage category, and there are notices in the waiting room explaining what these categories mean. However, in many other countries, including Australia, patients are usually not told what the process of triage means or what their allocated triage category is. If patients know this, they are then in a position to make an informed decision about whether to wait in the emergency department or to seek other medical attention.

We are aware that governments have target waiting times for each triage category and that these may be unrealistic. Patients continually state that not knowing how long they might wait is a major frustration. We found that once patients understood why they might face delays (e.g. because staff need to deal with more critical patients, such as cardiac arrests), their anxiety and frustration was reduced.

Explain Emergency Department Processes   We recommend that staff explain to patients what is likely to happen next. For example, staff should inform patients that they are likely to be visited by different doctors at unpredictable times and that they may be sent for X-rays or tests. In particular, clinicians should tell patients that although shifts may change while they are in the emergency department, handover processes ensure that the oncoming personnel will be fully briefed and that patients will receive continuity of care.

Provide Clinical Explanations   We recommend that clinicians provide clinical explanations of the emergency department patient's diagnosis and treatment plan. Wherever possible, we suggest that staff also explain the reasoning processes behind these. Evidence from patient complaint statistics suggests that providing useful explanations is vital to meeting patients' expectations of quality care (NSW Health Care Complaints Commission 2013) and vital for patient compliance with treatment.

7.2.3   Develop Effective Interdisciplinary Teamwork

Emergency departments are multidisciplinary worksites but the care they provide is not always interdisciplinary. Although we observed strong teamwork at one emergency department, at most of them we saw nurses sharing information with nurses, doctors with doctors—and very little cross-disciplinary interaction or collaboration. This lack of multidisciplinary culture and behaviour can lead to failures to exchange vital patient information. It can also be associated with poor levels of respect between the disciplines and therefore a working environment that is less harmonious and less cooperative than would be ideal in the emergency department context. We therefore recommend that emergency department training and handover procedures take into consideration ways to improve multidisciplinary collaboration.

7.2.4   Develop Cross-Cultural Communication Awareness and Strategies

In most countries around the world the population is culturally and linguistically diverse, and this diversity is reflected in patient presentations to emergency departments, as well as in the clinical and administrative staff of those departments. Modern day health care is a multilingual and multicultural reality. In addition, emergency departments have to use agency and locum staff on a regular basis, which increases staffing variation, unfamiliarity, and team performance. There are many older patients in emergency departments, who may also be seen as a specific cultural group with values, expectations, and specific healthcare communication needs which differ from those of younger patients.

While several staff demonstrated significant awareness of cross-cultural factors and communication strategies when dealing with patients of different backgrounds and ages, the findings from the research highlighted many challenges of communication between culturally diverse patients and clinicians. Patients and clinicians often experienced difficulty understanding overseas accents and intonation patterns. Local and overseas-trained clinicians can also sometimes have trouble understanding each other's medical framing and explanations.

We suggest it would be useful to orient all staff to the issues associated with dealing with diverse population groups. For example, staff could be coached in the need to avoid cultural stereotyping, to give clear (possibly also written) follow-up instructions, to avoid complex questions and culturally specific references to pain with older patients.

We recommend that all staff receive training on appropriate ways of treating and communicating with patients from diverse population groups, as well as ways of working with staff from culturally and linguistically diverse backgrounds.

7.2.5   Introduce More Effective and Durable Forms of Patient Records

Communicating in the emergency department will always involve a combination of spoken and written exchanges, with the role of written documentation playing a significant role from both a medicolegal and a clinical perspective (Eisenberg et al. 2005; Hobbs 2007; Slade et al. 2008). Although our study focused on spoken language in emergency departments, our data indicated that patients' written records were a potential source of miscommunication and risk.

In clinician–patient interactions, our consultation transcripts demonstrate that successive clinicians continually requestion patients, seeking information that has been previously documented in their notes. In clinician–clinician interactions, usually, senior clinicians have been 'told' about the patient's illnesses (Coiera et al. 2002) by junior clinicians, but often they do not have the time to read notes and case histories before they approach the bedside, and even if they have read them, they prefer to ask the patient for the information themselves. However, our transcript data (and interviews with patients) suggests that this is taxing and confusing for patients, especially if the information is already available in the patient's notes and/ or has been provided by the patient earlier on in the consultation.

Our interviews with clinicians and our examination of patients' medical records highlighted ongoing 'disconnects' between the ways that spoken and written communication were meant to support or complement each other in the emergency department. Particular problems included the legibility, accuracy, equivalence, and accessibility of written documentation, as explained by one senior registrar:

> No, I mean, this occurs frequently that notes are so poorly written that they're of no help at all. Because we often try and get an idea looking back to the previous notes, you know, what they came in with last time, that sort of stuff. Or, or even handing over from shift to shift, so the night resident hands over and we go look and often they're so useless you have to go back and take your notes again. And that may be for different reasons, it may be because they're completely illegible. Maybe because they're so short. We were taught in medical school a particular way to write notes, most people follow that. Some people choose not to follow that and that makes it very difficult. Some people are very scanty with their notes, they'll take a big history and have a lot more information and if you ask them the question they'll tell you but they don't write them down. And so it becomes very difficult. And sometimes you've got no idea from the notes what's actually gone on. And I think other people write their notes, not that they're sort of lying but they want their notes to fit a picture so actually they'll write something that's not quite actually as it happened. And I think that the notes should be a true representation of what happened. Even though it's never true because things get lost with every, every step of communication, but I think they should be aiming to be a true representation of what happened. If you want to then sum it up into something that fits a picture, that's fine but you need, you need to [have a record].

With the refinement and development of electronic health records, ways to reduce the mismatch between what is said and what is written down must be investigated. For example, some hospitals are implementing the recording of spoken handovers by doctors on their iPhones as they are occurring, and other hospitals are using iPads at the patient bedside for the clinicians to immediately write down the necessary patient or handover information. However, despite initiatives like this and millions being spent around the world on implementing electronic health records, in most countries electronic health record systems are still not sophisticated enough to be able to reduce the gap between the crucial spoken information about the patient and what is recorded in the patient's medical records.

7.2.6   Provide Training with Authentic Materials

Effective clinical communication is recognised by medical and nursing accreditation bodies as a core skill essential for ensuring quality and safety in health care. While most health education courses teach clinical communication, the quality and extent of course content, resources and teaching methods can vary greatly. Medical and nursing students are rarely exposed to authentic materials or teaching and learning approaches that address communication in high-risk settings such as emergency departments. We recommend that the teaching of clinical communication skills be based on the research that analyses and describes real clinician–patient communication, such as the data presented in our research.

A 'Communication for Health in Emergency Contexts' (CHEC) project has been funded by the Australian Learning and Teaching Council to do this. It has drawn on the authentic transcripts recorded in our research that this book is based on. It has used the material to develop an innovative multimedia learning resource for nursing and medical students. The materials and activities reflect the cultural and linguistic diversity that clinicians will encounter in emergencies. (Woodward-Kron et al. 2011).

7.2.7   Examine Communication in Clinical Handovers

Our research in emergency departments recognised that although effective clinician–patient communication is essential for quality patient care, handover communication between clinicians is also critical. Substantial international research has identified problems in clinical handover and shown that clinician to clinician communication practices are also instrumental in ensuring patient safety (Cooper et al. 2007; Finn 2008; Finn and Waring 2006; Risser et al. 1999; Sheehan et al. 2007). The levels and kinds of cooperation amongst clinicians (Sheehan et al. 2007), the mix of permanent versus agency and locum staff (Finn and Waring 2006), and professional rivalries (Finn 2008) all affect clinician teamwork and have been found to have a bearing on patient care and patient safety. Failure to achieve effective clinical handover is recognised by the World Health Organization as one of the five leading sources of clinical incidents (WHO 2008). Despite this recognition, there is little systematic empirical evidence about why these incidents occur, and there is no language research base upon which programs of improvement in handovers can be built.

As a follow-up to the emergency department research for this book, Diana Slade has led an extensive 3-year national Australian Research Council funded research project into communication in clinical handover, entitled Effective Communication in Clinical Handover, across four states of Australia (Eggins and Slade, forthcoming Eggins and Slade, 2012).

7.2.8   *Examine Continuity of Care from Discharge to the Community*

It was beyond the scope of this research to follow the patient from discharge back to the community—an essential component of the continuity of care—but it is an important complement to this research. The interactions between the clinicians and patients, as well as those between the clinicians in discharge handovers, are the final opportunity to make sure the patient and their carers and the relevant community clinicians are fully briefed on the diagnoses, treatment plan, and follow-up care. Misunderstandings or gaps in communication at the discharge stage are linked to nonadherence to treatment plans and subsequent adverse events, leading to rehospitalisation (see Chap. 1). A cross-disciplinary project with an international team led by Phillip Della and involving among others Diana Slade, Suzanne Eggins, and Roger Dunston is about to begin following three vulnerable groups of patients—elderly, mental health and paediatric—from the point of discharge to the community. The aim of this project is to improve patient safety outcomes by analysing and then enhancing communication practices during transition of care at discharge for high risk clinical populations.

7.3   Conclusion

We hope that this book will contribute to clinicians' and patients' awareness of some of the main disjunctions affecting emergency care delivery. Our study shows how the 'successful' combination of patient involvement in their care, effective medical diagnoses, nursing and systemic support make for safe and comfortable journeys for patients through the emergency department, and how unresponsive combinations result in patient dissatisfaction, incomprehension, or, at worst, critical incidents. Using ethnographic, sociolinguistic, and discourse analyses, we have described how information about each patient is gathered, interpreted, transmitted, and then acted upon. We are hoping that our findings and recommendations will lead to systemic improvements, by allowing stakeholders to make sense (Weick 1995) of their own and others' institutional behaviours. Studies such as this may not harbour immediate effect, but rendering these problems and challenges visible by engaging in cross-disciplinary research and by providing explicit communication frameworks is a step towards making health practice—and healthcare communication—more explicit and effecting change.

The organisational and contextual challenges facing emergency department clinicians and the spontaneous nature of spoken language render these communication practices as 'taken for granted' (Berger and Luckman 1967) and invisible. We hope by making these spoken communication practices explicit and visible that we can see the powerful role communication plays in safe and quality care.

References

Berger, P.L., & Luckmann, T. (1967). *The social construction of reality: A treatise in the sociology of knowledge*, Penguin Social Sciences. UK: Berger and Luckmann.

Coiera, E.W., Jayasuriya, R.A., Hardy, J., Bannan, A., Thorpe, M.E.C. (2002). Communication loads on clinical staff in the emergency department. *Medical Journal of Australia, 176,* 415–418.

Cooper, S., O'Carroll, J., Jenkin, A., Badger, B. (2007). Collaborative practices in unscheduled emergency care: Role and impact of the emergency care practitioner—qualitative and summative findings. *Emergency Medicine Journal, 24*(9), 625–629.

Eisenberg, E.M., Murphy, A.G., Sutcliffe, K., Wears, R., Schenkel, S., Perry, S., Vanderhoef, M. (2005). Communication in emergency medicine: Implications for patient safety 1. *Communication Monographs, 72,* 390–413. doi:10.1080/03637750500322602.

Finn, R. (2008). The language of teamwork: Reproducing professional divisions in the operating theatre. *Human Relations, 61*(1), 103–130.

Finn, R., & Waring, J. (2006). Organizational barriers to architectural knowledge and teamwork in operating theatres. *Public Money and Management, 9,* 117–124.

Hobbs, P. (2007). The communicative functions of the hospital medical chart. In R. Iedema (Ed.), *The discourse of hospital communication: Tracing complexities in contemporary health care organizations*. Houndmills: Palgrave Macmillan.

NSW Health Care Complaints Commission (2013) Annual Report 2012–2013.

Risser, D.T., Rice, M.M., Salisbury, M.L., Simon, R., Jay, G.D., Berns, S.D. (1999). The potential for improved teamwork to reduce medical errors in the emergency department. *Annals of Emergency Medicine, 34*(3), 373–383.

Sheehan, D., Robertson, L., Ormond, T. (2007). Comparison of language used and patterns of communication in interprofessional and multidisciplinary teams. *Journal of Interprofessional Care, 21(1), 17–30.*

Slade, D., Scheeres, H., Manidis, M., Iedema, R., Dunston, R., Stein-Parbury, J., Matthiessen, C., Herke, M., McGregor, J. (2008). Emergency communication: The discursive challenges facing emergency clinicians and patients in hospital emergency departments. *Discourse & Communication, 2,* 271–298. doi:10.1177/1750481308091910.

Stewart, M. (2001). Towards a global definition of patient centred care. *BMJ* (Clinical research ed.) *Care, 21*(1), 17-30.

Weick, K.E. (1995). *Sensemaking in organizations*. London: SAGE.

Woodward-Kron, R., Slade, D., Flynn, E., Stein-Parbury, J., Widin, J., Smith, L., Scheeres, H. (2011). Multimedia learning and teaching resources. Communication for Health in Emergency Contexts (CHEC): Teaching and learning resource for emergency department communication. Media learning and teaching resources, Final report. http://www.chec.meu.medicine.unimelb.edu.au/. Accessed March 2015.

World Health Organization (WHO) (2008). Action on patient safety: high 5s. At: http://www.who.int/patientsafety/implementation/solutions/high5s/ps_high5s_project_overview_fs_Oct_2011.pdf. Accessed 13 Oct 2013.

Index

© Springer-Verlag Berlin Heidelberg 2015
D. Slade et al., *Communicating in Hospital Emergency Departments*,
DOI 10.1007/978-3-662-46021-4